CKD STAGE 4

And

TYPE 2 DIABETES

COOKBOOK

Nutritious Low Sodium, Low Potassium, and Low Carb Recipes for Managing Kidney Disease and Blood Sugar Levels, with a 30-Day Meal Plan for Better Health

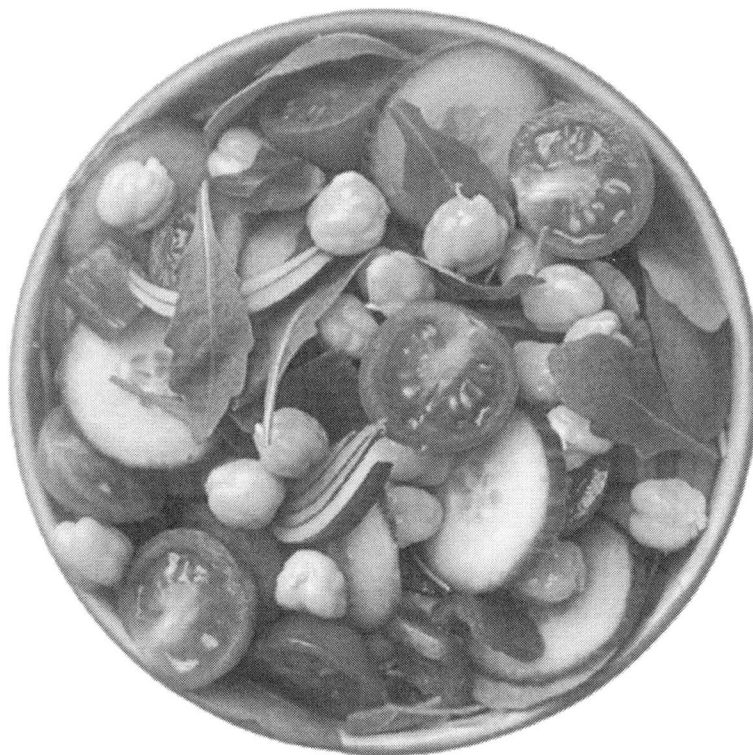

Dr. Maria Hall

COPYRIGHT

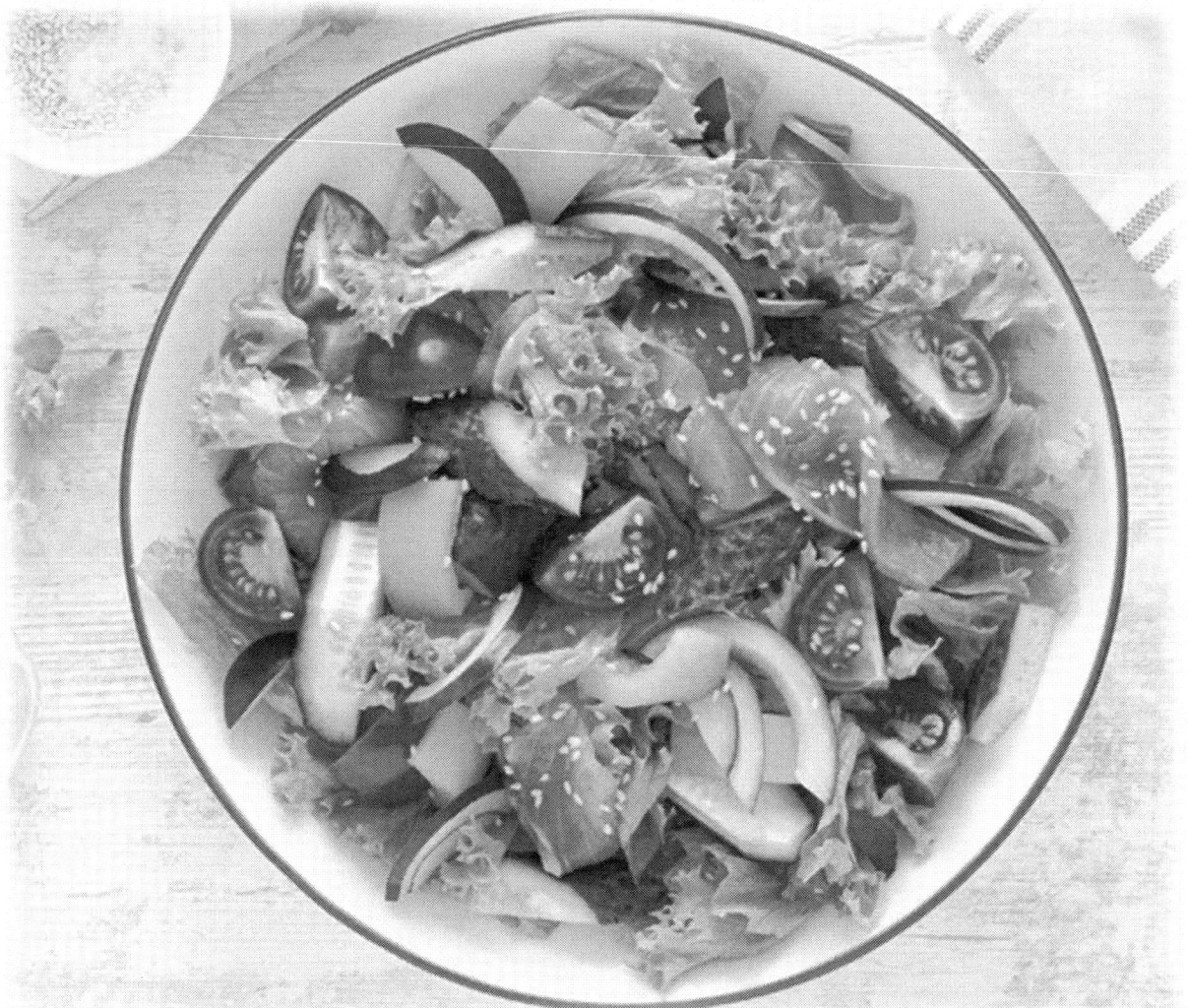

TABLE OF CONTENTS

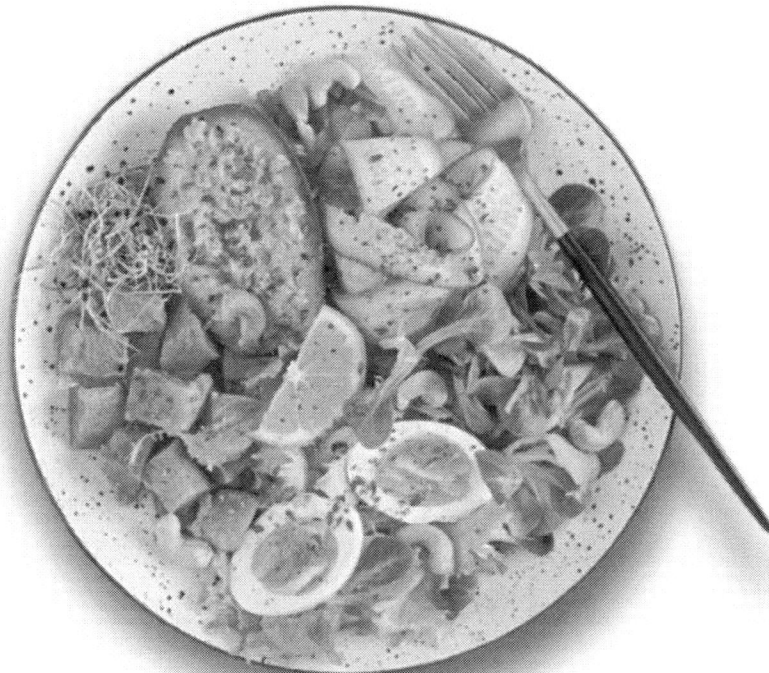

INTRODUCTION

Managing Type 2 Diabetes and Stage 4 Chronic Kidney Disease (CKD) can be difficult, particularly when it comes to meal planning. A careful dietary balance is necessary for these two disorders in order to preserve renal function and keep blood sugar levels steady. However, maintaining a healthy diet doesn't have to mean compromising on taste or pleasure.

The purpose of this CKD Stage 4 and Type 2 Diabetes Cookbook is to provide tasty, useful answers to your nutritional requirements. Every recipe is made with blood sugar control in mind and is low in salt, potassium, and phosphorus. Regardless of how long you have had these problems or how recently you were diagnosed, this cookbook offers recipes that can help you maintain your health and wellbeing.

This book is more than simply a compilation of recipes; it's a tool to help you live well and enjoy your food, even with dietary limitations, since it offers advice on portion sizes, component substitutions, and professional advice for managing both illnesses. Find meals that complement your lifestyle and provide you with the self-assurance to prepare meals with ease and provide your body with nourishment that promotes long-term health.

CHAPTER 1: UNDERSTANDING CKD STAGE 4 AND TYPE 2 DIABETES

Type 2 diabetes and chronic kidney disease (CKD) are two severe yet frequently related illnesses that have a major impact on the body's capacity to operate normally. When both are present, controlling them necessitates paying close attention to nutrition and lifestyle.

What is CKD Stage 4?

Chronic kidney disease (CKD) is characterized by a gradual deterioration in kidney function. By Stage 4, the kidneys' function has significantly declined, typically falling between 15% and 29% of its typical capacity. Because the kidneys can no longer filter waste, excess fluid, and toxins from the blood, the body now builds up poisonous substances. Poorly managed CKD Stage 4 can lead to renal failure (Stage 5), which requires dialysis or a kidney transplant.

For people with Stage 4 CKD, a strict diet is required to reduce the burden on their kidneys. This means avoiding foods that are heavy in sodium, potassium, and phosphorus while still ensuring that you are getting enough nutrition to maintain your health and energy levels.

What is Type 2 Diabetes?

In type 2 diabetes, the body either stops producing enough insulin to control blood sugar levels or grows resistant to it. Consistently elevated blood sugar levels over time might harm the kidneys as well as other bodily systems and organs. Since the kidneys' sensitive filtering units can be harmed by the ongoing stress of controlling high blood glucose, diabetes is really one of the main causes of chronic kidney disease (CKD).

Meal planning becomes much more difficult for people with both Type 2 Diabetes and Chronic renal Disease (CKD) because blood sugar levels and renal function must be balanced. While certain minerals must be consumed in moderation to preserve kidney health, carbohydrates must be closely watched to prevent blood sugar increases.

The Importance of a Balanced Diet

Diet is crucial for managing Type 2 Diabetes and Stage 4 CKD since it can reduce the disease's progression and enhance quality of life. A healthy diet can help keep blood sugar levels steady, lessen the strain on the kidneys, and avoid problems from both diseases.

Key aspects of this diet include:

- **Low Sodium:** Overconsumption of sodium damages kidneys by increasing blood pressure and causing fluid retention. Reducing sodium intake lessens the burden on the cardiovascular and renal systems.
- **Reduced Potassium and Phosphorus:** When kidney function is compromised, the body may accumulate high levels of potassium and phosphorus, which can result in harmful problems. Foods high in these minerals are minimized in a CKD-friendly diet.
- **Blood Sugar Control:** For people with Type 2 Diabetes, controlling carbohydrate intake is essential to avoiding blood sugar increases and reducing the chance of additional kidney damage.

IMPORTANCE OF DIET IN MANAGING BOTH CONDITIONS

One of the most effective ways to manage your health and stop further issues when you have both Type 2 Diabetes and Chronic Kidney Disease (CKD) Stage 4 is through food. Because diet has a direct impact on blood sugar regulation and renal function, it is important to pay close attention to what you eat in order to balance the nutritional requirements of these two disorders. The following explains why diet is so important for managing Type 2 Diabetes and Stage 4 CKD:

1. **Protecting Kidney Function**

The kidneys can no longer efficiently filter waste and extra fluid from the blood at Stage 4 of CKD because they are only operating at 15–29% of their full potential. An appropriately controlled diet can lessen kidney strain and stop additional damage. Important dietary objectives for kidney health consist of:

- **Limiting Sodium**: High blood pressure, fluid retention, and worsened renal function can all result from consuming too much sodium. Cutting less on salt lowers the risk of cardiovascular problems and protects the kidneys.
- **Controlling Potassium and Phosphorus**: Excess potassium and phosphorus cannot be filtered out by the kidneys at Stage 4, which might result in major health problems including weak bones or heart problems. These issues can be avoided with a diet low in phosphorus (limited dairy and nuts) and potassium (avoiding bananas and potatoes).

2. Managing Blood Sugar Levels

Stable blood sugar levels are essential for people with Type 2 Diabetes in order to avoid long-term issues, such as more kidney damage. A diet that is suitable for diabetics helps you:

- **Monitor Carbohydrate Intake**: Blood sugar levels are directly impacted by carbohydrates. Blood sugar levels can be maintained by eating regular servings of healthy grains, legumes, and vegetables with a low glycemic index (GI).
- **Choose Healthy Fats and Proteins**: It's crucial to choose healthy fats (like avocados and olive oil) and modest amounts of plant-based proteins to prevent renal overload while maintaining stable blood sugar levels because diets heavy in fat and protein can strain the kidneys.

3. Reducing the Risk of Complications

You can lower your risk of serious problems like renal failure, neurological damage, and cardiovascular disease by controlling your blood sugar levels and kidney function through food. High blood pressure, which is frequent in those with diabetes and chronic kidney disease, can also be managed with a well-balanced diet.

4. Maintaining Nutritional Balance

Managing two diseases that necessitate dietary restrictions makes it more difficult to meet your nutritional demands. To stay healthy and energized without making your situation worse, you must continue to consume enough calories, vitamins, and minerals. A customized nutrition plan can assist you in:

- **Avoid Malnutrition**: Malnutrition is a possibility with restricted diets, particularly when it comes to protein and calorie intake. You may make sure you obtain adequate nutrition while adhering to a diet that is suitable for people with CKD and diabetes by working with a healthcare professional or dietitian.
- **Incorporate Variety**: It might be challenging to stick to a diet that feels overly restrictive. Finding diabetic and kidney-friendly substitutes can allow you to continue enjoying a wide range of delectable dishes without feeling restricted.

5. Promoting Overall Health

A nutritious diet can help you control your blood pressure, cholesterol, and weight—all of which are critical for treating Type 2 Diabetes and Chronic Kidney Disease. Additionally, a well-balanced diet increases your energy, elevates your mood, and improves your general quality of life, which makes it simpler to manage your condition on a daily basis.

In conclusion, nutrition is crucial for controlling Type 2 Diabetes and Stage 4 CKD. It guarantees you receive the proper nutrients to maintain your health while lowering the risk of problems, controlling blood sugar, and protecting your kidneys. You may retain a higher quality of life and enhance your health results with the appropriate dietary plan.

NUTRITIONAL GUIDELINES: LOW SODIUM, POTASSIUM, AND PHOSPHORUS

Following certain dietary recommendations is crucial for people with Type 2 Diabetes and CKD Stage 4 in order to preserve renal function and keep blood sugar levels in check. Since the kidneys are currently unable to filter excessive amounts of salt, potassium, and phosphorus, it is especially crucial to concentrate on lowering intake of these minerals. Let's examine these rules in more detail:

1. Low Sodium Guidelines

Sodium, which is frequently present in processed foods and salt, can raise blood pressure and promote fluid retention, all of which place additional strain on the heart and kidneys. Limiting salt consumption is essential for controlling blood pressure, lowering edema, and delaying the progression of renal disease in Stage 4 of CKD. Controlling salt intake also supports heart health in those with Type 2 Diabetes, which is particularly crucial because diabetes raises the risk of heart disease.

Key Sodium Guidelines:

- **Recommended Intake:** Depending on the recommendations of your healthcare practitioner, try to consume no more than 1,500–2,000 mg of sodium daily.
- **Avoid Processed and Packaged Foods:** These frequently have high salt content. Be wary of processed meats, canned soups, freezer entrees, and snack items like chips.
- **Read Labels:** Always examine food labels for sodium content and look for goods that are low in sodium or sodium-free.
- **Use Herbs and Spices:** Use vinegar, lemon, garlic, fresh herbs, and spices to add flavor to your food instead of salt.

Foods to Avoid:

- Salted foods, such as crackers, pretzels, and chips
- Processed and canned meats (deli meats, bacon, sausages)
- Soups and sauces in packages
- Restaurant dinners and fast food

Foods to Include:

- Fresh fruits and vegetables (choose low-potassium varieties)
- Meals prepared at home with little to no salt
- Fresh poultry, fish, or meats (without salt)
- Whole grains such as oats and brown rice

2. Low Potassium Guidelines

Hyperkalemia, or dangerously high potassium levels, can result from the kidneys' inability to eliminate excess potassium from the blood in Stage 4 CKD. Symptoms of high potassium include heart failure, irregular heartbeats, and muscle weakness. Limiting potassium is therefore crucial. However, a balance is required because potassium is essential for heart and muscle function.

Key Potassium Guidelines:

- **Recommended Intake:** Limiting potassium intake to 2,000–3,000 mg daily is a basic recommendation that will be tailored by your healthcare practitioner based on your blood potassium levels.
- **Choose Low-Potassium Fruits and Vegetables:** It's crucial to select fruits and vegetables that are lower in potassium while still offering vital nutrients because not all of them are high in potassium.
- **Limit Potassium-Rich Foods:** Steer clear of foods like bananas, oranges, potatoes, and tomatoes that are known to contain high potassium levels.

Foods to Avoid:

- Oranges, bananas, kiwis, and cantaloupe
- Avocado, spinach, tomatoes, and potatoes
- Dried fruits, such as prunes and raisins
- Seeds and nuts

Foods to Include:

- Pineapples, grapes, berries, cherries, and apples
- Green beans, cabbage, cucumbers, lettuce, and cauliflower
- Pasta and white bread have less potassium than whole grains.
- Rice milk (a low-potassium alternative to milk)

3. **Low Phosphorus Guidelines**

Another mineral that the kidneys have trouble controlling at Stage 4 CKD is phosphorus. Because the body tries to make up for it by taking calcium from the bones, high blood phosphorus levels can weaken them and cause issues with the heart and bones. Keeping your phosphorus intake under control protects your heart and bones.

Key Phosphorus Guidelines:

- **Recommended Intake:** The recommended daily intake of phosphorus is often between 800 and 1,000 mg. Depending on your test findings, your healthcare provider will adjust this quantity.
- **Limit High-Phosphorus Foods:** These consist of processed foods with phosphorus additions, dairy products, some meats, nuts, and seeds.
- **Be Cautious with Packaged Foods:** Phosphorus additives found in many processed and packaged meals are rapidly absorbed by the body and increase phosphorus levels more readily than phosphorus found naturally in whole foods.

Foods to Avoid:

- Dairy goods (ice cream, yogurt, cheese, and milk)
- Peanut butter, seeds, and nuts
- Dark drinks, such as root beer and colas
- processed goods that contain phosphate additions (look for terms like "calcium phosphate" or "phosphoric acid" on labels).

Foods to Include:

- Alternatives to dairy milk (almond milk, rice milk)
- Vegetables that are fresh or just cooked
- Fresh poultry and meats (in moderation, without phosphates added)
- White rice, cornmeal, and refined grains are examples of low-phosphorus grains.

BALANCING BLOOD SUGAR WHILE PROTECTING KIDNEY HEALTH

Achieving the delicate balance between blood sugar control and renal function protection is crucial for managing both Type 2 Diabetes and Chronic renal Disease (CKD) Stage 4. Because the kidneys must filter waste and surplus nutrients and blood sugar levels must stay stable to stop further damage, both illnesses necessitate careful dietary monitoring. The following techniques can assist in balancing both:

1. Managing Carbohydrates to Control Blood Sugar

For people with Type 2 Diabetes, limiting carbohydrate intake is essential because they have a direct effect on blood sugar levels. It's crucial to strike a balance between this and the requirement to preserve kidney function. The secret is controlling portion sizes and selecting the appropriate kinds of carbs.

Tips for Managing Carbs:

- **Choose Low Glycemic Index (GI) Foods:** Low GI foods digest more slowly, which raises blood sugar levels gradually. These foods keep blood sugar levels steady without taxing the kidneys too much. Whole grains (like quinoa and barley), legumes (like lentils and chickpeas), and non-starchy vegetables (such leafy greens and cauliflower) are a few examples.
- **Avoid High-Glycemic Foods:** Fast blood sugar increases from high-GI foods might be especially dangerous for people with Type 2 Diabetes. Steer clear of refined carbs like white bread, pastries, sugary snacks, and sugary drinks.
- **Control Portion Sizes:** Overconsumption of even healthy carbohydrates can cause blood sugar levels to rise. To maintain stable blood sugar levels, use smaller plates and bowls, measure meals, and pay attention to portion sizes to prevent overindulging.

2. Incorporating Protein in Moderation

Although protein is necessary for good health, too much of it can strain the kidneys. A modest amount of protein is required for those with CKD Stage 4 in order to sustain body processes and avoid muscle loss, but too much protein can hasten renal deterioration. It's critical to maintain steady blood sugar levels when balancing protein intake.

Protein Guidelines:

- **Focus on Lean Protein Sources:** Select lean, premium proteins that don't put undue strain on the kidneys. These consist of fish, chicken without skin, and plant-based foods including lentils, beans, and tofu.

- **Avoid Excessive Animal Protein:** Excessive consumption of animal protein, particularly red and processed meats, might put more stress on the kidneys. When consuming red meat in meals, try to limit your intake and opt for smaller quantities.
- **Distribute Protein Throughout the Day:** To assist balance blood sugar and ease renal function, distribute protein equally among meals rather than taking big amounts in one sitting.

3. Limiting Sodium to Protect Kidney Health

One of the most crucial minerals to restrict while treating chronic kidney disease is sodium. Consuming too much sodium can cause renal damage, high blood pressure, and fluid retention. Limiting salt is also crucial for general heart health because individuals with Type 2 Diabetes are more likely to develop cardiovascular disease.

Sodium Guidelines:

- **Limit Processed and Packaged Foods:** Processed foods are frequently lacking in nutrients and heavy in salt. These foods can damage kidney function by increasing blood pressure and causing fluid retention. Steer clear of deli meats, freezer dinners, canned soups, and salty snacks.
- **Flavor with Herbs and Spices:** To flavor food without adding salt, use dried or fresh herbs such as rosemary, thyme, oregano, and basil. Great substitutes for salt include vinegar, lemon, garlic, and onion.
- **Monitor Labeling for Sodium Content:** When buying processed or packaged foods, look at the sodium content on the nutrition labels and, if you can, choose low-sodium or sodium-free options.

4. Managing Potassium and Phosphorus Intake

In order to preserve kidney health, controlling potassium and phosphorus levels is just as vital as maintaining blood sugar balance. High phosphorus can weaken bones and have an adverse effect on cardiovascular health, while excessive potassium can cause harmful side effects such cardiac arrhythmias.

Potassium Guidelines:

- **Choose Low-Potassium Fruits and Vegetables:** You should eat vegetables like green beans, lettuce, and cauliflower, as well as fruits like apples, berries, and grapes that are low in potassium. These choices give vital vitamins and minerals without putting too much potassium in the kidneys.
- **Limit High-Potassium Foods:** Foods high in potassium, such as bananas, oranges, potatoes, tomatoes, and dried fruits, should be avoided or consumed in moderation.

Phosphorus Guidelines:

- **Limit Phosphorus-Rich Foods:** Phosphorus is abundant in dairy products, nuts, seeds, and some meats, particularly processed meats. Limiting these items helps avoid phosphorus accumulation, which can cause problems with the heart and bones.
- **Avoid Phosphate Additives:** Foods containing added phosphorus, such processed and packaged foods, should be avoided as they frequently contain additives like "phosphoric acid."

5. Focusing on Healthy Fats

Although they are a necessary component of the diet, fats should be carefully chosen, particularly for people with diabetes and chronic kidney disease. For people with Type 2 Diabetes, heart health and blood sugar regulation are greatly enhanced by healthy fats.

Healthy Fat Sources:

- **Monounsaturated Fats:** Healthy fats found in nuts, avocado, and olive oil (in moderation) enhance kidney function and help balance blood sugar.
- **Omega-3 Fatty Acids:** Omega-3 fatty acids are abundant in plant-based foods like flaxseeds and walnuts, as well as fatty seafood like salmon, mackerel, and sardines. Because of their anti-inflammatory qualities, these fats may help maintain kidney health and enhance blood sugar regulation.
- **Avoid Trans Fats and Saturated Fats:** Reduce your intake of foods high in trans and saturated fats, such as packaged snacks, fried foods, and fatty red meat cuts, as they can worsen blood sugar problems and renal disease.

6. Staying Hydrated with the Right Fluids

Hydration is crucial, however people with Stage 4 CKD must carefully control their fluid intake, particularly if they have fluid retention. Maintaining adequate fluids promotes better kidney function and guards against dehydration, which raises blood sugar levels.

Hydration Guidelines:

- **Monitor Fluid Intake:** You might need to restrict how much fluid you drink, depending on what your doctor advises. Limiting fluid intake can help avoid renal strain in cases of fluid retention.
- **Choose Water or Low-Calorie Drinks:** The best hydration beverage is water, however low-calorie drinks like herbal teas can also be helpful. Steer clear of sugary drinks and sodas that might raise blood sugar levels.

- **Be Mindful of Electrolyte Imbalances:** Make sure you're not losing vital electrolytes like calcium, potassium, and salt when you change your fluid consumption. For kidney function and blood sugar regulation, electrolyte and fluid intake must be balanced.

Maintaining kidney health while controlling blood sugar necessitates a multifaceted strategy that takes into account the particular requirements of each disease. You may assist protect your kidneys while keeping your blood sugar levels steady by limiting sodium, potassium, and phosphorus, incorporating healthy fats, controlling your diet of carbohydrates, and limiting your intake of protein. To ensure optimum health and well-being, it's critical to collaborate with a healthcare professional or dietician to create a customized plan that meets your unique requirements.

CHAPTER 1: NAVIGATING THE DIET

WHAT TO EAT: APPROVED FOODS LIST

Choosing foods that balance blood sugar levels and safeguard kidney function is essential for controlling Type 2 Diabetes and Chronic Kidney Disease (CKD) Stage 4. Whole, minimally processed foods that supply vital nutrients without taxing the kidneys or raising blood sugar levels are the mainstay of the optimal diet for these disorders. A list of acceptable foods to include in your diet is provided below:

1. **Fruits (Low Potassium Options)**

Although fruits are an excellent source of fiber and vitamins, choosing the right ones is important to control potassium levels. Avoid foods that can raise blood sugar levels and choose fruits that are low in potassium.

Approved Fruits:

- Apples
- Berries (strawberries, blueberries, raspberries)
- Cherries
- Grapes
- Pears
- Pineapple
- Plums
- Peaches
- Watermelon (in moderation)

2. Vegetables (Low Potassium and Low Phosphorus)

In addition to being high in vitamins, minerals, and fiber, some vegetables are high in potassium, which can be harmful to those who have chronic kidney disease. Select kidney-friendly, low-potassium alternatives and steer clear of phosphorus-rich ones.

Approved Vegetables:

- Cauliflower
- Green beans
- Lettuce (romaine, iceberg)
- Cucumbers
- Bell peppers (red, green, yellow)
- Zucchini
- Cabbage
- Carrots
- Kale (in moderation)
- Asparagus

3. Whole Grains (Low Glycemic Index)

When taken in moderation, whole grains are good for the kidneys, help control blood sugar, and provide you energy. For blood sugar regulation, whole grains with a low glycemic index are preferable.

Approved Whole Grains:

- Quinoa
- Brown rice (in moderation)
- Barley
- Oats (steel-cut or rolled)
- Whole wheat pasta (in moderation)
- Millet
- Buckwheat
- Whole-grain bread (low-sodium, low-phosphorus)

4. Lean Proteins (Kidney-Friendly Options)

Maintaining muscle mass and general health requires protein, but too much protein can strain the kidneys. Select protein sources that are lean, high-quality, and easier for the kidneys to digest.

Approved Lean Proteins:

- Skinless chicken or turkey breast
- Fish (salmon, mackerel, sardines, cod)
- Tofu
- Tempeh
- Eggs (in moderation)
- Plant-based proteins (lentils, chickpeas, beans)
- Low-fat dairy (in moderation, depending on phosphorus levels)

5. Healthy Fats (Heart-Healthy Options)

Good fats promote general cardiovascular health and blood sugar stability. Select unsaturated fats that are good for renal health and diabetes.

Approved Healthy Fats:

- Extra virgin olive oil
- When eaten in moderation, avocados
- Nuts and seeds (little amounts of walnuts, flaxseeds, chia seeds, and almonds)
- Nut butters (without salt or sweetener)
- Fish high in fat, such as sardines, mackerel, and salmon

6. Dairy (Low Phosphorus and Low Sodium)

Although dairy products can be high in phosphorus, which may need to be controlled in CKD, they are a good source of protein and calcium. Select dairy products that are lower in salt and phosphorus.

Approved Dairy (in moderation):

- Rice milk (fortified with calcium and vitamin D) or unsweetened almond milk
- Plain, low-fat, phosphorus-controlled Greek yogurt
- Cottage cheese (small amounts, low in salt)

7. Beverages (Hydration Without Overload)

Although it's important to stay hydrated, people with CKD Stage 4 may have negative effects from consuming too much fluid. Select drinks that won't raise blood sugar levels and are good for your kidneys.

Approved Beverages:

- Hydration without extra sugars: water
- Teas made from herbs (like peppermint and chamomile)
- Iced tea without added sugar
- Coffee (in moderation, without extra sugar)
- Water with lemon or lime (no extra sugar)

8. Herbs and Spices (Natural Flavoring)

It is possible to improve flavor without impairing kidney function or raising blood sugar levels by substituting herbs and spices for salt or sodium-rich condiments.

Approved Herbs and Spices:

- Basil, parsley, oregano, thyme, rosemary, cilantro, and other fresh or dried herbs
- Spices (garlic powder, onion powder, paprika, cumin, turmeric, and cinnamon)
- Vinegar (balsamic, apple cider)
- Juice from lemons
- Pepper, black

9. Sweeteners (For Blood Sugar Control)

Although it's ideal to restrict additional sugars, people with diabetes can safely use several sugar alternatives. Select sweeteners that don't impact blood sugar levels and aren't high in calories.

Approved Sweeteners:

- Stevia
- Monk fruit sweetener
- Erythritol (in moderation)

You can protect your kidneys and maintain stable blood sugar levels while managing Type 2 Diabetes and CKD Stage 4 by include the aforementioned authorized foods in your diet. To make sure your dietary choices are suited to your individual needs, always get advice from a dietician or your healthcare professional.

FOODS TO AVOID

Avoiding items that can decrease kidney function, cause blood sugar spikes, and create other issues is essential while managing Type 2 Diabetes and Chronic Kidney Disease (CKD) Stage 4. To safeguard your kidneys, regulate blood sugar, and enhance general health, you should cut back on or completely avoid these meals.

1. High-Sodium Foods

Consuming too much sodium can damage renal function, increase blood pressure, and cause fluid retention. Limiting salt consumption is crucial to avoiding these problems.

Foods to Avoid:

- Processed meats (bacon, sausage, hot dogs, deli meats)
- Canned soups, broths, and sauces (unless labeled low-sodium)
- Packaged snack foods (chips, pretzels, salted popcorn)
- Frozen dinners and ready-to-eat meals
- Instant noodles and ramen
- Salted nuts and seeds
- Condiments like soy sauce, ketchup, and salad dressings (high in sodium)
- Pickled foods and olives

2. High-Potassium Foods

In CKD, the kidneys have difficulty eliminating excess potassium, which can cause cardiac issues, muscle weakness, and other dangerous side effects. Steer clear of foods high in potassium to maintain balanced levels.

Foods to Avoid:

- Bananas, oranges, and other high-potassium fruits (e.g., kiwi, melons, dried fruits)
- Potatoes (especially in large portions), sweet potatoes, and yams
- Tomatoes and tomato-based products (e.g., sauces, ketchup, salsa)
- Avocados
- Spinach, beet greens, and other leafy greens (high potassium in large servings)
- Dried beans, lentils, and peas (high potassium)
- High-potassium fruit juices (orange juice, prune juice, etc.)

3. High-Phosphorus Foods

An excess of phosphorus in the blood can cause cardiovascular and bone issues. Limiting meals high in phosphorus is crucial for maintaining kidney and bone health.

Foods to Avoid:

- Dairy products (milk, cheese, yogurt, ice cream)
- Processed meats (bacon, sausages, hot dogs)
- Nuts and seeds (almonds, walnuts, sunflower seeds)
- Nut butters (e.g., peanut butter, almond butter)
- Dark sodas (colas, root beer, etc.)
- Fast food (many contain added phosphorus)
- Packaged snacks (chips, crackers, and cookies with added phosphates)

4. Refined Carbohydrates and Sugary Foods

Blood sugar increases from refined carbs and sugary foods are dangerous for those with Type 2 Diabetes. To improve blood sugar regulation, these foods should be reduced or avoided.

Foods to Avoid:

- White bread, white rice, and white pasta
- Sugary cereals
- Pastries, cakes, cookies, and donuts
- Sweetened beverages (sodas, energy drinks, sweetened teas)
- Candy, chocolate, and other sugary snacks
- Ice cream, sweetened frozen desserts
- Granola bars with added sugars and syrups

5. Fried Foods and Trans Fats

Trans fats and fried foods can increase blood cholesterol and heart disease risk, which is already present in people with Type 2 Diabetes. Additionally, they lead to renal strain.

Foods to Avoid:

- Fried fast food (fried chicken, french fries, fried snacks)
- Fast food and takeout meals that are deep-fried
- Processed snack foods (chips, cookies, crackers with trans fats)
- Margarine, shortening, and partially hydrogenated oils
- Fried desserts like donuts and fritters

6. High-Sugar Alcoholic Beverages

Some people with Type 2 Diabetes may be able to drink alcohol in moderation, however sugary alcoholic beverages can cause blood sugar levels to spike quickly and lead to weight gain. Numerous alcoholic beverages are also harmful to renal health, especially when chronic kidney disease is progressed.

Foods to Avoid:

- Sweet wines (moscato, dessert wines)
- Sugar-sweetened beer and ciders
- Margaritas and piña coladas are examples of cocktails made with sweet mixers.
- Premade mixed beverages, which are frequently rich in salt and sugar

7. Artificial Sweeteners (In Excess)

When taken in excess, certain artificial sweeteners can have an adverse effect on renal function. They don't contain calories, but moderation is key.

Foods to Avoid:

- Artificially sweetened soft drinks and diet sodas (in excess)
- snacks and foods that contain artificial sweeteners (such as sucralose, aspartame, etc.)
- Desserts and candies without added sugar (use in moderation)

8. High-Fat Animal Products

Animal products high in fat can raise cholesterol and worsen cardiovascular issues, which puts those with Type 2 Diabetes at risk. When taken in excess, they can also strain the kidneys.

Foods to Avoid:

- Red meat (pork, lamb, and beef)
- Whole milk, full-fat cheese, and cream are examples of full-fat dairy products.
- Bologna, pepperoni, and salami are examples of processed meats.
- Poultry cuts that are high in fat, such as skin-on chicken or duck
- Fried poultry and meats (such as breaded meats and fried chicken)

9. Processed and Packaged Foods with Additives

Numerous processed meals include dangerous preservatives, chemicals, and toxic fats that can impair blood sugar, kidney function, and general health.

Foods to Avoid:

- Frozen dinners and microwaveable meals
- Canned vegetables with added salt

- Packaged snacks with artificial colors, flavors, and preservatives
- Pre-packaged deli meats and cheeses

By avoiding the foods mentioned above, you can protect your kidneys, maintain stable blood sugar levels, and better manage Type 2 Diabetes and CKD Stage 4. Rather, concentrate on wholesome, nutrient-dense foods that promote diabetic control and kidney function. To make sure your diet fits your unique health needs, it's always a good idea to speak with your doctor or nutritionist.

PORTION CONTROL AND MEAL TIMING

Meal timing and efficient portion control are essential management techniques for Type 2 Diabetes and Chronic Kidney Disease (CKD) Stage 4. They lessen kidney strain, stop blood sugar spikes, and enhance general wellness. You can better control your blood sugar levels and safeguard your kidney function by being mindful of when and how much you consume.

1. **The Importance of Portion Control**

Maintaining a healthy weight and regulating blood sugar both depend on portion control, which can lessen the strain on the kidneys. Consuming substantial amounts of meals high in calories or sugar can raise blood sugar levels and put more strain on the kidneys, which is crucial in Stage 4 of chronic kidney disease. Managing both illnesses requires an understanding of portion proportions for various dietary groups.

Tips for Portion Control:

- **Use smaller plates and bowls**: By giving the appearance of a fuller plate with fewer amounts, this helps people avoid overindulging.
- **Measure serving sizes**: Learn the typical serving sizes for the various dietary groups, such as 3 ounces of lean protein and 1/2 cup of cooked vegetables.
- **Avoid second servings**: If you have already consumed a sufficient amount of food, try not to return for more.
- **Read food labels**: Check the serving size on packaged foods whenever you can, and steer clear of items that are high in harmful fats, sugar, or sodium.
- **Use hand portions**: Using your hand as a reference is a quick and simple method of portion management (e.g., a serving of protein should be around the size of your palm).

2. **Balancing Macronutrients**

At each meal, it's critical to balance the macronutrients (fats, proteins, and carbohydrates) for the best blood sugar and renal control. This lowers the chance of kidney damage and helps maintain stable blood sugar levels.

- **Carbohydrates**: Select complex carbohydrates (whole grains, non-starchy veggies, etc.) that have a low glycemic index. Reduce your intake of processed foods and refined sugars that raise blood sugar levels quickly.
- **Protein**: When it comes to protein consumption in CKD, moderation is essential. While too little protein might result in malnutrition, too much protein can overload the kidneys. Prioritize lean proteins (such as fish, poultry, and tofu) and abide by the daily protein intake guidelines set forth by your healthcare practitioner.
- **Fats**: Limit saturated and trans fats, which can raise cholesterol and lead to cardiovascular problems, and include heart-healthy fats, such as those found in almonds, avocados, and olive oil.

3. Meal Timing and Frequency

The number and timing of meals are essential for controlling blood sugar levels and avoiding undue renal strain. Equally distributing meals and snacks throughout the day keeps blood sugar levels steady and keeps the kidneys from being overloaded with too much food to process all at once.

Meal Timing Tips:

- **Eat smaller, more frequent meals**: Aim for four to six smaller meals or snacks throughout the day rather than three large ones. This gives the kidneys a reasonable amount of food to digest and aids in blood sugar regulation.
- **Avoid large meals late at night**: Large meals consumed late at night can cause sleep disturbances and poor blood sugar regulation, both of which can be detrimental to kidney health. Try to finish your meal two to three hours before going to bed.
- **Eat consistent meals at regular intervals**: To maintain constant blood sugar levels, try to eat at similar times each day. Your body maintains insulin sensitivity thanks to this constancy.
- **Plan meals around physical activity**: Meals should be timed before or after physical activity if you regularly exercise to avoid blood sugar swings. A balanced breakfast one to two hours prior to exercise, for instance, might assist fuel the body and avoid hypoglycemia, or low blood sugar, during or after exercise.

4. Managing Blood Sugar Spikes

Controlling Type 2 Diabetes requires avoiding blood sugar rises. These surges can be avoided and more stable blood sugar levels can be maintained by the time of your meals and the kinds of foods you eat.

Strategies to Prevent Blood Sugar Spikes:

- **Pair carbs with protein or healthy fats**: To slow down digestion and lessen the effect on blood sugar, balance carbs with protein or healthy fats.
- **Avoid sugary beverages**: Energy drinks, sodas, and sweetened juices are examples of sugary beverages that can quickly raise blood sugar levels. Instead, choose low-calorie drinks like water or unsweetened teas.
- **Limit high-carb foods**: Select fruits, vegetables, and whole grains that have a low glycemic index. Steer clear of processed carbohydrates and refined grains as they might cause sharp increases in blood sugar.
- **Stay hydrated**: Water consumption throughout the day supports renal function and blood sugar regulation. Higher blood sugar levels and lower renal health can result from dehydration.

5. Special Considerations for CKD Stage 4

Kidney function deteriorates when chronic kidney disease (CKD) worsens, necessitating a restriction in meals heavy in salt, potassium, and phosphorus. In order to avoid kidney damage, portion control becomes even more important.

CKD-Specific Tips:

- **Limit fluid intake**: Fluid retention may become a problem in severe chronic kidney disease. Monitor your fluid intake and refrain from consuming too many drinks, particularly those high in sugar or caffeine, if your doctor has recommended it.
- **Monitor potassium and phosphorus**: Foods high in potassium and phosphorus should be avoided since they can build up in the blood when kidney function is compromised. For precise instructions, speak with your healthcare provider.
- **Track protein intake**: In Stage 4 CKD, your doctor could advise decreasing protein consumption to lessen renal strain. To reduce renal workload, concentrate on eating high-quality proteins and space out your protein intake throughout the day.

6. Practical Tips for Managing Portion Control and Meal Timing

- **Use a food journal**: To stay aware of what you're eating and how it affects your blood sugar and kidney function, keep a record of your meals and portion amounts.
- **Pre-portion meals**: To prevent overindulging, prepare and portion your meals ahead of time. Making better decisions and managing nutrient balance can also be aided by this.
- **Eat slowly and mindfully**: Avoid hurrying through meals and pay attention to your body's signals of hunger and fullness. Eating mindfully helps improve digestion and avoid overindulging.

- **Get support**: Consult a registered dietitian or other healthcare professional who specializes in chronic kidney disease and diabetes if you struggle to manage portion control and meal time. They can assist you in developing a food plan according to your requirements.

Meal timing and portion control are crucial for the management of Type 2 Diabetes and Stage 4 CKD. You can help keep blood sugar levels steady, safeguard renal function, and enhance general health by eating smaller, more balanced meals at regular intervals. Your eating habits will be in line with your health objectives if you work with a dietician or healthcare professional to create a customized meal plan.

CHAPTER 2: MEAL PLANNING FOR CKD STAGE 4 AND TYPE 2 DIABETES

BUILDING A BALANCED PLATE FOR CKD STAGE 4 AND TYPE 2 DIABETES MANAGEMENT

Managing Type 2 Diabetes and Stage 4 Chronic Kidney Disease (CKD) both depend on eating a balanced plate. By eliminating excessive amounts of salt, potassium, and phosphorus that could damage your kidneys or alter blood sugar levels, a balanced plate makes sure you are getting the proper amounts of carbohydrates, proteins, fats, and veggies.

Maintaining good blood sugar levels, lessening kidney strain, and promoting general health are all made possible by a well-balanced plate. Here's how to create a balanced plate for the best blood sugar and kidney care:

1. **Half of the Plate: Non-Starchy Vegetables**

The majority of your plate should be made up of non-starchy vegetables. These vegetables are a great way to control blood sugar and safeguard renal function because they are low in calories, carbs, sodium, and potassium (if picked correctly). They are abundant in vitamins, minerals, and fiber—all of which are critical for preserving general health.

Examples of Non-Starchy Vegetables:

- Leafy greens (e.g., spinach, kale, lettuce)
- Broccoli, cauliflower, and Brussels sprouts
- Bell peppers, cucumbers, and zucchini
- Carrots, green beans, and asparagus
- Mushrooms, eggplant, and tomatoes (in moderation)

- Cabbage, onions, and garlic

Benefits:

- **Blood Sugar Control**: These veggies, which are high in fiber, assist to stabilize blood sugar levels by slowing down the absorption of sugars.
- **Kidney Protection**: Non-starchy veggies are kidney-friendly options for CKD Stage 4 since they are low in potassium and salt.
- **Nutrient-Rich**: Vitamin C, folate, potassium, and other vital vitamins and minerals are found in these veggies and are crucial for good health.

2. One-Quarter of the Plate: Lean Proteins

Protein is necessary for muscle mass maintenance and body repair, however in Stage 4 CKD, it's crucial to limit protein consumption to prevent kidney overload. Select lean proteins with less saturated fat and phosphorus. Depending on your unique health situation and the advice of your physician, your protein requirements may change.

Examples of Lean Proteins:

- Poultry without skin (turkey or chicken)
- Seafood and fish (such as shrimp, tilapia, and salmon)
- Plant-based proteins like tempeh or tofu
- Lean beef or pork cuts, such as tenderloin and sirloin
- Moderate consumption of eggs
- Cheese with less fat (if your doctor recommends it)

Benefits:

- **Blood Sugar Control**: Protein slows down the breakdown of carbohydrates, which helps to balance blood sugar.
- **Kidney Protection**: Compared to high-fat animal proteins, lean proteins are less likely to cause renal strain.
- **Muscle Maintenance**: For people with CKD who may have muscle wasting, protein is essential for maintaining muscle mass.

3. One-Quarter of the Plate: Whole Grains or Healthy Carbohydrates

Although complex carbohydrates with a low glycemic index are crucial for people with Type 2 Diabetes to prevent blood sugar increases, carbohydrates are still a vital source of energy. Because they are high in fiber and affect blood sugar levels more gradually, whole grains and other healthful carbohydrates are a wonderful option.

Examples of Whole Grains and Healthy Carbohydrates:

- Brown rice, quinoa, and farro
- Whole wheat pasta and bread (look for 100% whole wheat)
- Oats and barley
- Sweet potatoes (in moderation, depending on potassium levels)
- Legumes (beans, lentils, chickpeas) (moderate portions)

Benefits:

- **Blood Sugar Control**: Whole grain fiber slows the absorption of sugar, avoiding sharp rises in blood sugar.
- **Kidney Protection**: Whole grains offer a well-balanced carbohydrate source that is low in potassium and salt.
- **Digestive Health**: A high fiber content promotes intestinal health and facilitates digestion.

4. Healthy Fats (Optional but Recommended in Moderation)

Your meals should contain healthy fats, but in moderation. Fats improve cell activity, aid in vitamin absorption, and give off energy. Choose unsaturated fats since they lower cholesterol and are good for the heart. Enhancing insulin sensitivity, which can aid in the management of Type 2 Diabetes, is another benefit of these lipids.

Examples of Healthy Fats:

- Olive oil, avocado oil, and coconut oil (used in moderation)
- Nuts and seeds (e.g., almonds, chia seeds, flaxseeds)
- Nut butters (unsweetened and in moderation)
- Avocados
- Fatty fish (e.g., salmon, mackerel, sardines)

Benefits:

- **Heart Health**: Both CKD and diabetes benefit from healthy fats' ability to reduce inflammation and minimize the risk of cardiovascular disease.
- **Blood Sugar Control**: In order to promote more stable blood sugar levels, fats aid in slowing the absorption of carbs.

- **Kidney Protection**: Kidney function can be preserved and inflammation can be decreased with the help of unsaturated fats.

5. Optional: Small Serving of Fruits (With Caution for CKD)

Fruits are a great source of vitamins, minerals, and antioxidants, but in Stage 4 CKD, they should be ingested in moderation because of their potassium level. Choose fruits with less potassium and concentrate on those that don't significantly impact blood sugar levels.

Examples of Low-Potassium Fruits:

- Apples, pears, and peaches
- Berries (e.g., strawberries, blueberries, raspberries)
- Grapes and cherries
- Pineapple (in moderation)
- Watermelon (in moderation)

Benefits:

- **Blood Sugar Control**: Fruits with a low glycemic index assist avoid sudden rises in blood sugar.
- **Antioxidant-Rich**: Antioxidants, found in fruits like berries, aid in shielding cells from oxidative damage.
- **Kidney Health**: Fruits low in potassium lower the chance of blood potassium accumulation, which is crucial for CKD.

6. Beverages: Focus on Hydration

The greatest beverage for sustaining kidney function and staying hydrated is water. Those without CKD should try to drink lots of water throughout the day, even if some persons with the disease need to decrease their fluid consumption. Be cautious with sugary or high-sodium beverages, as they can negatively impact blood sugar and kidney health.

Examples of Hydrating Beverages:

- Water (with or without lemon)
- Unsweetened herbal tea (e.g., peppermint, chamomile)
- Black coffee (in moderation)

Benefits:

- **Kidney Function**: By preventing dehydration and aiding in the removal of toxins, staying hydrated promotes kidney health.
- **Blood Sugar Control**: Blood sugar levels can be maintained by consuming water and unsweetened liquids.

Creating meals that are high in non-starchy veggies, lean proteins, whole grains, healthy fats, and carefully chosen fruits is the key to managing Type 2 Diabetes and Chronic Kidney Disease (CKD) Stage 4. You may support kidney function, control blood sugar, and keep up a balanced, nutrient-dense diet by adhering to this recommendation. Meal time and portion control are also essential for making sure your plate supports your health objectives and maintains appropriate blood sugar and renal function. For individualized advice based on your particular requirements, always speak with your healthcare professional or dietician.

CALORIC AND NUTRIENT CONSIDERATIONS

Both blood sugar regulation and kidney health protection depend on calorie and nutrient intake management.

Caloric Intake:

- Adjust your calorie intake according to your weight, degree of activity, and current health.
- To ease the burden on the kidneys and enhance blood sugar regulation, maintain a healthy weight.
- To aid with portion management and avoid overeating, eat smaller, more frequent meals.

Nutrient Considerations:

- **Carbohydrates**: To control blood sugar, choose foods that are high in fiber and low in glycemic.
- **Proteins**: Prioritize lean proteins, but keep an eye on your consumption to prevent renal overload.
- **Fats**: Consume heart-healthy fats sparingly to preserve kidney and heart health.
- **Vitamins and Minerals**: Limit potassium, sodium, and phosphorus intake while making sure you are getting enough of the necessary nutrients.

TIPS FOR EATING OUT AND STAYING ON TRACK

Managing Type 2 Diabetes and Stage 4 CKD might make eating out difficult, but you can still enjoy meals out without sacrificing your health if you plan ahead and practice mindfulness. The following useful advice can help you keep on course:

1. Plan Ahead

- **Review the menu online**: A lot of eateries make their menus and nutritional data available online. To choose healthier options that fit your dietary requirements, go over them beforehand.
- **Ask about modifications**: Never be scared to ask for changes, such as removing high-potassium items, dressing on the side, or grilling rather than frying.

2. Control Portions

- **Order smaller portions**: Select smaller servings, including lunch-sized meals or appetizers. A to-go box is always an option, and you can store half for later.
- **Share dishes**: Overeating can be avoided and portion sizes can be managed by eating meals with friends or family.

3. Focus on Vegetables

- **Make vegetables the star**: Choose recipes that include vegetables that aren't starchy. Request additional vegetables on the side if they aren't included in the meal.
- **Avoid creamy, buttery sides**: Select vegetables that are grilled or cooked without extra fats instead.

4. Choose Lean Proteins

- **Select grilled or baked options**: Choose lean foods like chicken, fish, or tofu that are grilled, baked, or broiled rather than ones that are fried or breaded.
- **Watch the sodium**: Due to their high sodium content, request sauces and dressings on the side.

5. Skip Sugary Beverages

- **Choose water or unsweetened beverages**: Avoid sugary drinks that can raise blood sugar levels by sticking to water, sparkling water, or unsweetened tea.

6. Limit High-Kalorie Foods

- **Avoid heavy, fried, or sugary dishes**: Fried, highly sauced, or sugary foods should be avoided since they raise blood sugar levels and can cause renal strain.
- **Ask for nutrient-dense sides**: Limit starchy alternatives like white rice or potatoes and go for nutritious grains like quinoa or brown rice.

7. Pay Attention to Sodium and Potassium

- **Request less salt**: The sodium content of many restaurant dishes is high. Avoid adding salt at the table and request that your dish be cooked with less salt.
- **Monitor potassium**: Foods high in potassium, such as potatoes, tomatoes, or bananas, should be avoided, particularly if you need to regulate your potassium levels.

8. Mind Your Timing

- **Avoid late-night dining**: The management of renal disease and diabetes can be impacted by eating large meals late at night since it can alter blood sugar levels and interfere with sleep.

These guidelines can help you manage your Type 2 Diabetes and Stage 4 CKD while still enjoying eating out. Never forget to let your waitress know about any dietary restrictions you may have, and don't be afraid to change your order.

CHAPTER 3: COOKING TIPS FOR MANAGING CKD AND DIABETES

HOW TO REDUCE SODIUM WITHOUT LOSING FLAVOR

Because too much salt can strain the kidneys and raise blood pressure, lowering sodium is essential for controlling Type 2 Diabetes and CKD Stage 4. However, flavor does not have to be sacrificed in order to reduce sodium intake. The following techniques will help you improve the flavor of your food while controlling your sodium intake:

1. Use Fresh Herbs and Spices

- **Herbs**: Vibrant flavors can be added without adding salt by using fresh herbs like oregano, thyme, rosemary, cilantro, parsley, and basil.
- **Spices**: Try a range of spices, including ginger, turmeric, paprika, cumin, and garlic powder. These improve taste and provide potential health advantages.

- **Citrus**: Zest from lemons, limes, or oranges gives foods without salt a boost of brightness and freshness.

2. Experiment with Vinegars and Acids

- **Vinegar**: In order to balance the flavors of marinades, sauces, and roasted vegetables, balsamic, red wine, apple cider, or white vinegar can add depth and tang.
- **Lemon and Lime Juice**: Squeezing lemon or lime juice into food can add a cool tang that cuts down on salt.

3. Use Salt-Free Seasoning Blends

- A variety of handmade or store-bought salt-free seasoning blends can enhance the flavor of your food. Seek out mixes that contain dried veggies, herbs, and spices, like:
  - Italian seasoning
  - Cajun seasoning
  - Curry powder
  - Chili powder

4. Roast or Grill for Intensified Flavor

- **Roasting or grilling vegetables, meats, and fish** can concentrate their flavors naturally. The natural sweetness and savory characteristics are enhanced by the caramelization process, which facilitates salt reduction.

5. Use Umami-Rich Foods

- **Umami** is the savory flavor that brings out the best in flavors. Umami-rich foods can compensate for a lack of salt:
  - Tomatoes (with CKD in moderation)
  - Portobello and shiitake mushrooms, for example
  - Nutritional yeast (a fantastic alternative to dairy and salt for a cheesy taste)
  - Seaweed (wakame or nori, for example)
  - Aged cheeses (if your doctor has approved them)

6. Limit Processed Foods

- Hidden salt is frequently present in packaged and processed meals. You have more control over how much salt is used in your meals when you cook fresh foods at home.

7. Use Low-Sodium or No-Salt Added Alternatives

- Select canned foods, broths, sauces, and condiments that are **low in sodium** or have no added salt. Tomato paste, canned beans, and sodium-free or low-sodium soy sauce are all available for kidney health.

8. Add Sweetness to Balance Salt

- A dish's salty qualities can be balanced with a little sweetness from things like honey, maple syrup, or stevia, which lessens the need for additional salt.

By employing these strategies, you may lower your sodium consumption without compromising taste, which will help you manage Type 2 Diabetes and Stage 4 CKD while still indulging in filling, delectable meals.

SUBSTITUTING HIGH-POTASSIUM INGREDIENTS

Controlling potassium consumption is crucial for people with Type 2 Diabetes and Stage 4 CKD because too much potassium can harm the kidneys and impair heart function. Thankfully, you can replace high-potassium items in your meals in a number of ways without sacrificing flavor. Here are a few useful alternatives:

1. Potatoes

Although potatoes contain a lot of potassium, there are many other foods that might have comparable flavors and textures.

Substitutes:

- **Sweet Potatoes** (in moderation, as they still contain some potassium)
- **Cauliflower**: The texture of mashed cauliflower might be comparable to that of mashed potatoes.
- **Turnips**: As a low-potassium substitute for potatoes, these can be roasted or mashed.
- **Butternut Squash**: A mildly sweet substitute that works well for roasting or pureeing.

2. Tomatoes

Because tomatoes are high in potassium, you can control your potassium consumption by using them instead.Because tomatoes are high in potassium, you can control your potassium consumption by using them instead.

Substitutes:

- **Red Bell Peppers**: These have less potassium and a pleasant, slightly acidic taste.
- **Cucumbers**: Excellent as a low-potassium, refreshing addition to salads and sandwiches.
- **Zucchini**: Zucchini has a mild flavor and can be roasted in place of tomatoes or added to stir-fries and sauces.

3. Bananas

Although bananas are recognized for having a high potassium content, other fruits have comparable sensations without being very high in potassium.

Substitutes:

- **Apples**: A lower potassium substitute that is crispy and high in fiber.
- **Pears**: These are lower in potassium and have a sweetness and texture that is comparable to bananas.
- **Berries**: Antioxidant-rich and low in potassium are raspberries, blueberries, and strawberries.
- **Watermelon**: A fruit that is lower in potassium and hydrating.

4. Avocados

Avocados are rich in nutrients, but they also contain a lot of potassium.

Substitutes:

- **Olives**: A fantastic way to add creaminess or use in salads and spreads.
- **Hummus**: Hummus, which is made from chickpeas, has a creamy texture and contains less potassium.
- **Tofu**: A plant-based protein that can give salads and smoothies a creamy texture.

5. Spinach

Although spinach has a lot of potassium, it can be substituted with leafy greens that have less potassium.

Substitutes:

- **Lettuce**: In salads, romaine or iceberg lettuce work well in place of spinach.
- **Kale**: Kale can be included to smoothies or salads because it has less potassium.
- **Arugula**: A somewhat spicy substitute that works well in salads and wraps.

6. **Dried Fruits (e.g., Raisins, Dates)**

Potassium can be found in concentrated form in dried fruits.

Substitutes:

- **Fresh Apples or Pears**: Without the high potassium level of dried fruits, offer a natural sweetness.
- **Berries**: Berries, whether fresh or frozen, are a nutrient-dense choice that doesn't contain too much potassium.
- **Peaches or Plums**: These are lower in potassium and can be added to snacks or desserts.

7. **Orange Juice**

Due to its high potassium content, orange juice can be replaced with other drinks.

Substitutes:

- **Apple Juice**: A low-potassium, pleasant substitute for orange juice.
- **Cranberry Juice**: Cranberry juice that hasn't been sweetened can have a sour taste and have less potassium.
- **Lemonade (unsweetened)**: offers a fruity substitute without the high potassium content.

You can lower your potassium intake while still eating delicious, filling meals that help control Type 2 Diabetes and Chronic Kidney Disease Stage 4. For individualized advice on potassium limits and appropriate substitutes, always speak with your doctor or dietician.

SMART SUGAR SUBSTITUTES FOR DIABETICS

Living with Type 2 Diabetes requires careful blood sugar management, and avoiding spikes while yet sating your sweet tooth can be achieved by choosing wise sugar substitutes. You can enjoy sweet sensations without sacrificing your health by using these great sugar substitutes:

1. Stevia

Stevia is a sugar substitute made from plants that has no calories and doesn't cause blood sugar levels to rise. Only a little amount is required because it is far sweeter than sugar.

Benefits:

- No effect on blood sugar and no calories.
- natural, made from the plant stevia.
- It may have a faint aftertaste, but it's good for baking and cooking.

2. Erythritol

For diabetics, erythritol is a suitable option because it is a sugar alcohol that has little to no impact on blood sugar levels.

Benefits:

- Almost minimal calories and no effect on blood sugar.
- It works nicely in baked items and tastes a lot like sugar.
- To improve flavor balance, it is frequently used with other sweets.

3. Monk Fruit Sweetener

Another natural, calorie-free sweetener is monk fruit, which is far sweeter than sugar and requires very little. The blood sugar levels are unaffected.

Benefits:

- No blood sugar spikes or calories.
- made from a natural alternative—monk fruit extract.
- For a more well-rounded flavor, it is frequently combined with other sweeteners.

4. Xylitol

With a lower glycemic index than ordinary sugar, xylitol is a sugar alcohol that has less of an effect on blood sugar levels.

Benefits:

- 40% fewer calories than sugar, roughly.
- An alternative to sugar in recipes at a 1:1 ratio.
- It is a fantastic option for dental health since it helps prevent cavities.

5. Allulose

Allulose is a low-calorie sweetener that has a similar taste and consistency to sugar but fewer calories. It little affects blood sugar levels.

Benefits:

- minimally affects blood sugar levels and is low in calories.
- It has a texture and sweetness comparable to sugar and can be used in baking and cooking.
- less uncomfortable for the stomach than certain other sugar alcohols since it is more easily absorbed by the body.

6. Sucralose (Splenda)

Sucralose is a common artificial sweetener that has no calories and no effect on blood sugar levels. It is also several times sweeter than sugar.

Benefits:

- No impact on blood glucose levels and no calories.
- It can be used in baking and cooking because it is heat-stable.
- widely accessible and frequently found in prepared goods.

7. Agave Syrup

The agave plant is the source of agave syrup, which is a suitable choice for diabetics because it has a lower glycemic index than sugar.

Benefits:

- You need less because it's sweeter than sugar.
- reduced glycemic index, which causes blood sugar levels to climb more slowly.
- Perfect for cold dishes and drinks.

8. Coconut Sugar

Coconut sugar has a lower glycemic index and is less processed than ordinary sugar.

Benefits:

- includes trace levels of minerals and vitamins.
- lower than refined sugar in terms of glycemic index.
- Although it works well in baked items and drinks, it should still be used sparingly.

9. Date Sugar

Natural sugars, fiber, and antioxidants can be found in date sugar, which is prepared from dried and crushed dates.

Benefits:

- Packed with minerals and fiber, it's a healthier substitute for ordinary sugar.
- Although it still has some effect on blood sugar, it has a lower glycemic index than refined sugar.
- It works best when baked or cooked to provide a caramel-like flavor.

10. Yacon Syrup

The root of the yacon plant is used to make yacon syrup, which has a lower glycemic index and prebiotics to help maintain digestive health.

Benefits:

- lower in calories than sugar and with a low glycemic index.
- includes the prebiotic fiber inulin, which may help to support digestive health.
- Perfect for pouring over porridge or yogurt.

You can still enjoy sweet foods and beverages while improving blood sugar control by using these clever sugar replacements. Before adding new sweeteners to your diet, always with your doctor or nutritionist, particularly if you are worried about how they might impact your particular medical requirements.

BATCH COOKING AND FREEZING MEALS FOR CONVENIENCE

For people with Type 2 Diabetes and CKD Stage 4, batch cooking and storing meals is a terrific way to save time, maintain healthy eating habits, and provide convenience. You may simply follow your dietary recommendations and lessen the temptation to make unhealthy choices by preparing and storing meals in advance. Here's how to efficiently prepare meals in bulk and freeze them:

1. Plan Your Meals

- **Create a Meal Plan**: Organize your weekly meals according to your nutritional requirements, emphasizing ingredients that are low in salt, potassium, and diabetes. Pick foods that freeze well, such as casseroles, stews, soups, and grain-based dishes.
- **Batch Cooking Staples**: Make bigger quantities of adaptable staples that can be used in a variety of meals throughout the week, such as veggies, lean proteins (chicken, turkey, and tofu), and whole grains (quinoa, brown rice).

2. Choose Freezer-Friendly Recipes

Certain recipes are better at freezing than others. Choose foods that maintain their flavor and texture after freezing, like:

- **Soups and Stews**: Lean proteins and veggies are used to make many low-sodium soups and stews that freeze nicely.
- **Casseroles**: Freezing works best for casseroles that are high in veggies and low in salt, potassium, and phosphorus.
- **Grain Bowls**: Prepare grains such as brown rice or quinoa in advance and put them into freezer-safe containers so they can be combined with vegetables and proteins.

3. Portion Control

- **Pre-portion Meals**: Meals should be portioned into containers once they are cooked. This facilitates portion management and makes it simple to grab a meal when you're pressed for time.
- **Use Freezer Bags**: To save room and cut down on waste, think about using freezer bags for soups, sauces, or grain-based dishes. To facilitate stacking and speedy thawing, place bags flat in the freezer.

4. Label and Date Your Meals

- **Label Containers**: Always write the dish's name and the cooking date on the label. This guarantees that you consume the food within a safe window of time, which is usually three to six months for the majority of frozen dinners.
- **Use a Meal Rotation System**: Make careful to use older frozen foods first by rotating your meals. By doing this, food waste is reduced.

5. Proper Freezing Techniques

- **Cool Meals Before Freezing**: To keep ice crystals from forming and to preserve the food's texture, let meals drop to room temperature before freezing.
- **Use Airtight Containers**: To avoid freezer burn and maintain the food's flavor and texture, use freezer bags or airtight containers.
- **Avoid Freezing Certain Foods**: Certain items, such cooked eggs, dairy-based sauces, and vegetables with a high water content, like cucumber and lettuce, don't freeze well.

6. Thaw and Reheat Safely

- **Thaw in the Refrigerator**: Placing frozen foods in the refrigerator overnight is the safest way to thaw them. If you're pressed for time, you can also utilize your microwave's defrost mode.
- **Reheat Thoroughly**: To eliminate any microorganisms and guarantee food safety, reheat meals until the internal temperature reaches 165°F (74°C).

7. Meal Prep for Convenience

- **Snack Packs**: For convenient access, prepare tiny, snack-sized quantities of fruits, vegetables, or nuts and freeze them.
- **Breakfast Options**: For convenient morning meals, make breakfast dishes like egg muffins or overnight oats ahead of time, portion them up, and freeze them.

8. Make It a Family Activity

- **Get Help**: Include family members in meal preparation and freezing in bulk. It guarantees that everyone gets access to wholesome meals and speeds up and improves the process.

In addition to saving time, batch cooking and freezing meals also makes it simpler to follow your Type 2 Diabetes and CKD Stage 4 diet. Making your meals in advance will help you feel less stressed and resist the need to reach for harmful snacks. Additionally, you can be sure that your meals are nourishing and in line with your health objectives.

CHAPTER 4: MAINTAINING A HEALTHY LIFESTYLE

EXERCISE AND MOVEMENT FOR CKD AND TYPE 2 DIABETES

Exercise is essential for the management of Type 2 Diabetes and Stage 4 Chronic Kidney Disease (CKD). It lowers the risk of problems, maintains a healthy weight, improves quality of life, and improves general health. Exercise must be approached cautiously, though, to prevent blood sugar swings and kidney strain. Here's how to safely and successfully add movement and exercise to your routine:

1. Consult Your Healthcare Provider

Given the severity of diabetes and Stage 4 CKD, it's crucial to speak with your healthcare physician before starting any fitness program to be sure the activities you have planned are safe. They can offer tailored advice depending on your blood sugar regulation, kidney function, and present state of health.

2. Focus on Low-Impact Exercise

Type 2 diabetes and chronic kidney disease (CKD) can damage joint health and energy levels, so it's critical to emphasize low-impact workouts that are less taxing on the body while still having a positive health impact.

Examples:

- **Walking**: One of the greatest workouts for diabetics and persons with chronic kidney disease. You may complete it at your own time, and it's simple and accessible.
- **Swimming**: enhances cardiovascular health and strength while offering a full-body workout with no joint strain.
- **Cycling**: Cycling, whether indoors or out, is a fantastic way to strengthen your legs and heart.
- **Yoga**: In addition to helping with blood sugar regulation and renal function, gentle yoga can aid with flexibility, balance, and stress reduction.
- **Tai Chi**: A low-impact workout that emphasizes deliberate, slow motions that can help preserve flexibility, lower stress levels, and enhance balance.

3. Strength Training

Increasing insulin sensitivity, controlling blood sugar levels, and gaining muscle mass can all be facilitated by strength exercise. But pay attention to the frequency and level of intensity of your strength training.

Examples:

- **Resistance Bands**: Band-based low-resistance workouts are excellent for increasing strength without overtaxing the body.
- **Bodyweight Exercises**: Muscles can be strengthened with easy workouts like modified push-ups, lunges, and squats that don't require a lot of equipment.
- **Light Dumbbells**: Light weights can aid in improving insulin sensitivity, increasing metabolism, and toning muscles if your doctor gives the all-clear.

4. Aerobic Exercise

Exercises that increase lung capacity, lower blood pressure, and strengthen the heart include brisk walking, cycling, and swimming. Frequent aerobic exercise is particularly crucial for managing diabetes since it enhances insulin sensitivity and blood sugar regulation.

How to Start:

- As your endurance increases, progressively extend the duration of your aerobic workout from ten to fifteen minutes at a time.
- Over the course of at least three days a week, try to get in at least 150 minutes of moderate-intensity aerobic exercise (like brisk walking or cycling) or 75 minutes of strenuous exercise (like running).

5. Monitor Blood Sugar Levels

Monitoring your blood sugar levels before, during, and after exercise is crucial since activity can cause blood sugar levels to vary. By doing this, you can steer clear of hypoglycemia, or low blood sugar, and hyperglycemia, or excess blood sugar.

Tips:

- **Before Exercise**: Before beginning your workout, eat a little snack if your blood sugar is less than 100 mg/dL.
- **During Exercise**: In the event that your blood sugar falls, keep a fast-acting carbohydrate on hand, like glucose tablets.

- **After Exercise**: After exercising for 30 to 60 minutes, check your blood sugar again to be sure it's within a healthy range.

6. Stretching and Flexibility

Including stretching in your routine can help you become more flexible, avoid injuries, and relax your tense muscles. Additionally, stretching reduces stress, which is advantageous for the management of both diabetes and chronic kidney disease.

Suggestions:

- To keep your flexibility, do some light stretches both before and after your workouts.
- Incorporate stretches for the main muscular groups, particularly the arms, legs, and lower back.

7. Listen to Your Body

Don't overdo it and always pay attention to your body. Stop and speak with your doctor before continuing if you feel any pain, lightheadedness, shortness of breath, or discomfort when exercising.

8. Stay Consistent

The secret to reaping the rewards of exercise is consistency. Maintaining a regular exercise regimen can be difficult at first, but it will help you better control the symptoms of CKD and diabetes. Make an effort to include little amounts of activity in your everyday routine, such as standing while working, walking short distances, or using the stairs.

9. Incorporating Movement into Daily Life

Seek ways to enhance your daily activity if formal exercise seems too time-consuming or difficult:

- After meals, take quick walks to help control blood sugar levels.
- While watching TV or conversing on the phone, stand or move around.
- As you watch your favorite shows, stretch or perform some gentle yoga.

10. Rest and Recovery

Regular exercise is vital, but it's also critical to take breaks and give your body time to heal. Don't overdo it because both Type 2 Diabetes and Chronic Kidney Disease can produce weariness. Strive for a well-rounded schedule that includes enough days off in between harder workouts.

You may control your diabetes, preserve kidney function, and enhance your general health by adopting these lifestyle changes and workouts. Maintaining strength, vitality, and long-term heath requires regular exercise and mobility. To develop a safe and efficient fitness program for your particular condition, always get advice from your healthcare professional.

HYDRATION TIPS AND FLUID MANAGEMENT

For people with Type 2 Diabetes and Stage 4 Chronic renal Disease (CKD), maintaining adequate hydration is essential because it helps control blood sugar, preserve renal function, and avoid consequences from dehydration. Fluid intake must be carefully controlled, though, as too much fluid will strain the kidneys further and too little fluid might cause dehydration. The following are essential fluid management techniques and hydration advice for both conditions:

1. Understand Your Fluid Restrictions

It's critical to keep an eye on your fluid consumption when you have Stage 4 CKD to prevent renal overload. Depending on your particular condition, kidney function, and any other medical concerns, your healthcare professional will advise you on the appropriate amount of liquids to eat each day.

- **Fluid Restrictions**: In order to avoid edema or fluid retention, some people with CKD Stage 4 may need to restrict their fluid consumption. It's critical to adhere to your nephrologist's precise advice.
- **Fluid Recommendations for Diabetes**: Staying hydrated is crucial for Type 2 Diabetes in order to get the best blood sugar control. Blood sugar levels might rise as a result of dehydration, making diabetes management more difficult.

2. Drink Water as the Primary Beverage

The greatest way to stay hydrated without increasing your intake of calories, sugar, or sodium is to drink water.

- **Tip**: To remind yourself to stay hydrated during the day, keep a water bottle with you. Instead of consuming huge amounts at once, sip tiny amounts on a regular basis.
- **Infuse Water for Flavor**: Slices of lemon, lime, cucumber, or mint can be added to plain water to add taste without adding sugar if it seems too bland.

3. Monitor Electrolyte Balance

Electrolyte abnormalities, particularly with potassium, sodium, and phosphorus, can happen in CKD. Excessive fluid intake can affect these electrolyte levels, so it's important to balance your hydration with appropriate food choices.

- **Potassium and Sodium**: Keep an eye on your salt and potassium intake because these electrolytes might impact blood pressure and kidney function. Unless prescribed by your physician, choose low-sodium diets and stay away from potassium-rich drinks like fruit juices.
- **Use Electrolyte Drinks Carefully**: Certain electrolyte beverages may include excessive amounts of potassium or sugar. Choose low-potassium, sugar-free beverages if you're using these, and be sure they're safe for you by speaking with your doctor.

4. Hydrate with Diabetic-Friendly Beverages

Drinking sugar-free beverages to stay hydrated is essential for persons with Type 2 Diabetes to control their blood sugar levels.

- **Herbal Teas**: Herbal teas without added sugar, including chamomile, peppermint, or ginger tea, can be a terrific way to remain hydrated and have a relaxing beverage without causing blood sugar levels to rise.
- **Diluted Fruit Juices**: If you like fruit juice, dilute it with water to cut down on the amount of sugar. Before including them into your diet, choose low-potassium juices or obtain your doctor's consent.
- **Sugar-Free Drinks**: Sugar-free flavored water or sparkling water with a lemon twist are excellent substitutes for sugary beverages.

5. Avoid Excessive Caffeine and Alcohol

- **Caffeine**: As a diuretic, too much caffeine can make you need to urinate more frequently and perhaps cause dehydration. Reduce the amount of caffeinated drinks you consume, such as tea, coffee, and soda.
- **Alcohol**: It's recommended to drink alcohol sparingly or not at all because it can cause dehydration and alter blood sugar levels, particularly if you have diabetes or kidney problems.

6. Monitor for Signs of Dehydration

Understanding the symptoms of dehydration is critical to the management of Type 2 Diabetes and Chronic Kidney Disease. Dehydration symptoms include:

- Dry mouth or throat
- Fatigue or dizziness
- Dark yellow urine or decreased urination
- Headache or confusion

Increase your fluid intake and get advice from your healthcare professional if you have any symptoms of dehydration.

7. Eat Water-Rich Foods

You can increase your hydration by consuming meals high in water in addition to drinking fluids. These foods are low in calories and sugar, add extra water, and are easy on the kidneys.

Examples:

- **Cucumbers**: Ideal for remaining hydrated, it has a high water content and a low potassium concentration.
- **Watermelon**: A pleasant and hydrating choice that is suitable for moderate consumption.
- **Cantaloupe**: This fruit is also hydrating and has less potassium than other fruits like oranges or bananas.
- **Celery** is a fantastic low-calorie snack with a high water content.

8. Space Out Fluid Intake

Spread out your fluid intake throughout the day rather than guzzling a lot at once. This lowers the chance of fluid retention and helps prevent overtaxing your kidneys.

- **Small Sips**: Instead than consuming huge amounts at once, take tiny sips frequently throughout the day.
- **Timing**: To give your kidneys time to process and get rid of extra fluid, drink fluids early in the day. Reducing evening urine can be achieved by avoiding excessive fluid intake right before bed.

9. Adjust for Exercise and Heat

You might need to change how much liquids you consume if you exercise or are in hot conditions. It's crucial to stay hydrated, but in moderation, as heat and exercise can increase fluid loss through perspiration.

- **Pre-Exercise Hydration**: Maintain your hydration levels by drinking water both before and after exercise.
- **Post-Exercise**: Hydrate with water or a sugar-free electrolyte drink after working out to restore fluids without raising blood sugar levels.

10. Work with a Dietitian

See a nutritionist with expertise in diabetes and chronic kidney disease for individualized hydration plans. They can offer tailored advice depending on your medical condition, prescription drugs, and particular hydration needs.

You can enhance blood sugar regulation, support kidney function, and avoid consequences from Type 2 Diabetes and Chronic Kidney Disease by carefully controlling your fluid and hydration consumption. To make sure you're drinking enough water to support your general health and wellbeing, always heed the recommendations of your healthcare team.

STRESS MANAGEMENT TECHNIQUES FOR CKD AND TYPE 2 DIABETES

For people with Type 2 Diabetes and Stage 4 Chronic Kidney Disease (CKD), stress management is crucial. Blood sugar regulation and renal function can both be adversely affected by prolonged stress. It can aggravate the course of both illnesses and result in higher blood pressure and blood sugar levels. By putting stress management strategies into practice, one can lessen stress, enhance general wellbeing, and promote improved health outcomes. The following are some practical methods for managing stress:

1. Mindfulness and Meditation

Being in the present moment is the main goal of mindfulness and meditation techniques, which lower tension and encourage relaxation.

- **Breathing Exercises**: Breathing deeply and slowly can help you relax and reduce tension by triggering the parasympathetic nervous system. Spend a few minutes every day practicing diaphragmatic or deep breathing.
- **Mindfulness Meditation**: Sit quietly for ten to fifteen minutes every day and concentrate on your breathing, your feelings, or a positive statement. This technique can ease anxiety and promote mental calmness.
- **Guided Meditation**: For guided meditation sessions, use applications or videos found online. For novices, these can provide structure and assistance.

2. Physical Activity and Exercise

Frequent exercise is very helpful in treating Type 2 Diabetes and Chronic Kidney Disease (CKD) and is a natural stress reducer. The body's natural stress-relieving hormones, endorphins, are released when you exercise.

- **Gentle Exercise**: Take part in low-impact exercises like yoga, swimming, or walking to relieve tension without overtaxing your body.
- **Stretching**: Include stretching activities in your regular routine to increase flexibility and relax muscles, which will lessen stress and physical strain.
- **Tai Chi or Qi Gong**: These simple mind-body exercises, which emphasize awareness, breathing, and controlled movement, can help people relax and cope with stress.

3. Relaxation Techniques

Stress can be lessened and the body's natural relaxation response can be triggered with the use of relaxation practices.

- **Progressive Muscle Relaxation (PMR)**: PMR entails tensing and then relaxing the body's muscular groups. This method can help you relax and release bodily stress.
- **Visualization**: Imagine yourself in a serene, tranquil setting, such a forest or beach. Stress and anxiety can be lessened with the use of this mental images.
- **Soothing Music**: Your body and mind can feel calmed when you listen to relaxing music. Select soothing melodies and slow-paced music.

4. Healthy Sleep Habits

Good sleep hygiene should be prioritized because stress and sleep loss frequently coexist.

- **Establish a Sleep Routine**: To control your sleep cycle, go to bed and wake up at the same time every day, including on the weekends.
- **Create a Relaxing Sleep Environment**: Make sure your bedroom is quiet, cool, and dark. Don't use devices an hour or more before bed, including phones and TVs.
- **Limit Caffeine and Sugar**: Caffeine and sugary foods and beverages should be avoided in the evening since they can disrupt your sleep.

5. Time Management and Organization

Stress can be exacerbated by feelings of overwhelm. You might feel more in control and less stressed if you practice effective time management.

- **Prioritize Tasks**: Prioritize the most crucial activities and divide the larger ones into smaller, more doable steps. This will lessen the sensation of being overburdened.
- **Set Realistic Goals**: Establish attainable objectives and acknowledge your progress. Don't hold yourself to too many unattainable standards.
- **Delegate Responsibilities**: To lessen your workload and stress, assign responsibilities to others if at all possible.

6. Social Support

You can manage stress better if you have a solid support network. Your emotional burden can be lessened by talking to people about your experiences and feelings.

- **Talk to Loved Ones**: Talk about your feelings and worries with loved ones, friends, or a support group. Talking about your stress can sometimes make you feel understood and heard.

- **Join a Support Group**: Seek for in-person or online support groups for those with Type 2 Diabetes or Chronic Kidney Disease. Making connections with people who are aware of your difficulties can offer both practical advice and emotional support.
- **Spend Time with Pets**: Research indicates that interacting with pets helps reduce stress. Spend time with your pet and find solace in their companionship if you have one.

7. Hobbies and Leisure Activities

You can effectively divert your attention from tension and encourage relaxation by partaking in activities you enjoy.

- **Creative Activities**: Painting, drawing, knitting, and crafts are examples of hobbies that can be soothing and therapeutic.
- **Reading or Watching Movies**: Take a mental vacation from everyday worries by losing yourself in a good book or movie.
- **Gardening**: It has been demonstrated that spending time in outdoors and caring for plants lowers stress levels.

8. Professional Support

Stress can occasionally become too much to handle on your own. Additional support may be obtained by seeking expert assistance.

- **Therapy or Counseling**: A therapist can offer you coping mechanisms and assist you in examining the root causes of your stress. Anxiety and stress can frequently be effectively managed using cognitive behavioral therapy, or CBT.
- **Stress Management Classes**: Seek out online or local courses that provide emotional support and stress-reduction strategies.

9. Laughter and Humor

By lowering cortisol (the stress hormone) and producing endorphins, laughter has been demonstrated to lower stress and elevate mood. You may lighten the mood of your day by incorporating comedy.

- **Watch Comedies**: To improve your mood and calm your mind, watch comedic TV series, films, or stand-up comedy.
- **Spend Time with Fun People**: Be in the company of loved ones who enliven your life and make you laugh.

10. Healthy Nutrition

Stress management is significantly aided by eating a well-balanced diet. Consuming foods high in nutrients can help your body cope with stress.

- **Eat Balanced Meals**: To prevent blood sugar swings brought on by stress, concentrate on eating a diet high in vegetables, whole grains, lean meats, and healthy fats.
- **Limit Caffeine and Sugar**: These can lead to energy crashes and elevated stress levels. Instead, choose water and herbal teas.
- **Stay Hydrated**: Drink plenty of water throughout the day because dehydration can exacerbate stress.

You may lessen the negative effects of stress on your health and wellbeing by incorporating these stress-reduction strategies into your daily routine. Early stress detection and proactive stress management are crucial, particularly for people with CKD and Type 2 Diabetes. Discovering what works for you, whether it be through social support, exercise, or relaxation techniques, can have a big impact on how you feel.

RECIPES

CHAPTER 5: BREAKFAST RECIPES

1. LOW-SODIUM VEGGIE SCRAMBLE

Servings: 2

Prep Time: 10 min

Cook Time: 10 min

Total Time: 20 min

Ingredients:

- 4 large egg whites
- ½ cup of chop-up spinach
- ½ cup of diced bell pepper
- ¼ cup of chop-up onion
- 1 tbsp olive oil
- ¼ tsp black pepper
- Fresh herbs (parsley or chives) for garnish

Instructions:

1. In a non-stick skillet, flame the olive oil over medium heat.
2. Sauté the bell peppers and chop up onions for three to four minutes or until tender.
3. Cook the spinach for a further one to two min or until it wilts.
4. Add the egg whites, season with black pepper, and Cook the eggs by gently scrambling the mixture.
5. Garnish with fresh herbs and serve warm.

Nutrition Info (per serving):

Calories: 150

Protein: 12g

Carbohydrates: 5g

Fat: 10g

Sodium: 80mg

Potassium: 300mg

2. CINNAMON OATMEAL WITH BERRIES

Servings: 2

Prep Time: 5 min

Cook Time: 10 min

Total Time: 15 min

Ingredients:

- 1 cup of rolled oats
- 2 cups of water
- ½ tsp cinnamon
- ½ cup of mixed berries (blueberries, raspberries)
- 1 tbsp chia seeds (non-compulsory)
- 1 tsp sugar-free sweetener (non-compulsory)

Instructions:

1. Raise water or almond milk to a boil in a medium saucepan.
2. Turn down the heat to low and add the oats. Simmer, stirring periodically, for 5 to 7 min.
3. Add the chia seeds (if using) and cinnamon and stir.
4. Take off the heat and, if you'd like, garnish with a mixture of berries and sugar.
5. Warm up and serve.

Nutrition Info (per serving):

Calories: 200

Protein: 5g

Carbohydrates: 35g

Fat: 3g

Sodium: 10mg

Potassium: 200mg

3. HIGH-PROTEIN BREAKFAST MUFFINS

Servings: 6 muffins

Prep Time: 15 min

Cook Time: 20 min

Total Time: 35 min

Ingredients:

- 6 large egg whites
- ½ cup of diced mushrooms
- ½ cup of diced zucchini
- ¼ cup of diced onions
- ¼ cup of shredded low-fat cheese
- 1 tbsp olive oil
- ¼ tsp black pepper
- Fresh parsley for garnish

Instructions:

1. Lightly oil a muffin tray and preheat the oven to 350°F.
2. In a skillet, range the olive oil over medium heat. Sauté the onions, zucchini, and mushrooms for approximately five minutes or until tender.
3. Whisk the egg whites and black pepper in a large bowl. Add cheese and sautéed vegetables and stir.
4. Divide the mixture evenly among the muffin pans.
5. The egg muffins should be set after 15 to 20 minutes of baking.
6. Serve after adding some fresh parsley as a garnish.

Nutrition Info (per muffin):

Calories: 80

Protein: 10g

Carbohydrates: 3g

Fat: 3g

Sodium: 90mg

Potassium: 150mg

4. HERB-INFUSED EGG WHITE FRITTATA

Servings: 4

Prep Time: 10 min

Cook Time: 15 min

Total Time: 25 min

Ingredients:

- 8 large egg whites
- 1 cup of chop-up kale
- ½ cup of diced tomatoes
- ¼ cup of chop-up fresh basil
- 1 tbsp olive oil
- ½ tsp dried oregano
- ¼ tsp black pepper

Instructions:

1. Set the oven's temperature to 350°F.
2. In a medium ovenproof skillet, flame the olive oil over medium heat. Sauté the tomatoes and greens for three to four min.
3. Whisk the egg whites, fresh basil, oregano, and black pepper in a bowl.
4. Transfer the egg mixture to the veggie skillet. Cook for two to three min or until the edges begin to set.
5. The frittata should be cooked brown on top after 10 min of baking in the oven.
6. Cut into slices and warm up.

Nutrition Info (per serving):

Calories: 100

Protein: 12g

Carbohydrates: 4g

Fat: 4g

Sodium: 60mg

Potassium: 250mg

5. DIABETIC-FRIENDLY SMOOTHIE BOWL

Servings: 2

Prep Time: 10 min

Total Time: 10 min

Ingredients:

- 1 cup of unsweetened almond milk
- ½ cup of frozen strawberries
- ½ cup of frozen blueberries
- 1 tbsp chia seeds
- 1 tbsp almond butter
- ½ tsp vanilla extract
- Toppings: split almonds, fresh berries, and coconut flakes (non-compulsory)

Instructions:

1. Almond milk, chia seeds, almond butter, blueberries, frozen strawberries, and vanilla essence should all be mixed in a blender until smooth.
2. Transfer the smoothie mixture into two bowls.
3. Garnish with fresh berries, coconut flakes, and split almonds if preferred.
4. Serve right away.

Nutrition Info (per serving):

Calories: 180

Protein: 6g

Carbohydrates: 20g

Fat: 9g

Sodium: 50mg

Potassium: 220mg

6. LOW-POTASSIUM BREAKFAST CASSEROLE

Servings: 4

Prep Time: 15 min

Cook Time: 30 min

Total Time: 45 min

Ingredients:

- 6 large egg whites
- 1 cup of chop-up zucchini
- ½ cup of diced red bell pepper
- ½ cup of diced onion
- 1 cup of chop-up cauliflower
- ½ cup of shredded low-fat cheese (non-compulsory)
- 1 tbsp olive oil
- ¼ tsp black pepper
- 1 tsp dried thyme

Instructions:

1. Butter a casserole dish lightly and set the oven to 350°F.
2. In a skillet, flame the olive oil over medium heat. Sauté the red bell pepper, cauliflower, zucchini, and onions for 5 to 7 min or until tender.
3. Whisk the egg whites, dried thyme, and black pepper in a dish. Add the sautéed vegetables and stir.
4. Fill the casserole dish with the mixture. If using, top with shredded cheese.
5. Set the eggs in the oven for 25 to 30 minutes.
6. Before slicing and serving, allow the casserole to cool for a few min.

Nutrition Info (per serving):

Calories: 160

Protein: 12g

Carbohydrates: 6g

Fat: 9g

Sodium: 80mg

Potassium: 210mg

7. CHIA PUDDING WITH ALMOND MILK

Servings: 2

Prep Time: 5 min

Total Time: 5 min (+ 4 hrs or overnight to set)

Ingredients:

- 2 cups of unsweetened almond milk
- ¼ cup of chia seeds
- 1 tsp vanilla extract
- 1 tbsp sugar-free sweetener (non-compulsory)
- Fresh berries for topping (non-compulsory)

Instructions:

1. In a medium bowl, mix almond milk, chia seeds, vanilla extract, and sweetener (if using).
2. To avoid clumping, let the mixture settle for five minutes before whisking it again.
3. Cover the bowl and refrigerate for at least four hours or overnight to allow the chia seeds to absorb the liquid and thicken.
4. If preferred, garnish with fresh berries and serve.

Nutrition Info (per serving):

Calories: 120

Protein: 4g

Carbohydrates: 8g

Fat: 9g

Sodium: 100mg

Potassium: 180mg

8. WHOLE WHEAT TOAST WITH AVOCADO AND EGG

Servings: 1

Prep Time: 5 min

Cook Time: 5 min

Total Time: 10 min

Ingredients:

- 1 slice whole wheat bread
- ½ ripe avocado, mashed
- 1 large egg
- 1 tsp olive oil
- ¼ tsp black pepper
- ¼ tsp paprika (non-compulsory)

Instructions:

1. Bake the whole wheat bread until it turns golden.
2. Flame the olive oil in a skillet over medium temperature and cook the egg until it's done.
3. On top of the toasted bread, spread mashed avocado.
4. Sprinkle paprika (if used) and black pepper on top of the fried egg.
5. Serve on the spot.

Nutrition Info (per serving):

Calories: 250

Protein: 9g

Carbohydrates: 20g

Fat: 16g

Sodium: 140mg

Potassium: 450mg

9. SUGAR-FREE BANANA PANCAKES

Servings: 2

Prep Time: 10 min

Cook Time: 10 min

Total Time: 20 min

Ingredients:

- 1 ripe banana, mashed
- 2 large egg whites
- ¼ cup of almond flour
- 1 tsp baking powder
- 1 tsp vanilla extract
- ½ tsp cinnamon
- 1 tbsp sugar-free syrup (non-compulsory)

Instructions:

1. Put the ripe banana in a medium basin and mash.
2. Add the almond flour, baking powder, egg whites, cinnamon, and vanilla essence. Smoothly whisk.
3. Adjust the heat to medium in a non-stick skillet. To create tiny pancakes, pour the batter.
4. Cook for 2–3 minutes on each side or until browned and cooked through.
5. If desired, top with sugar-free syrup.

Nutrition Info (per serving):

Calories: 150

Protein: 8g

Carbohydrates: 20g

Fat: 5g

Sodium: 120mg

Potassium: 200mg

10. BLUEBERRY PROTEIN SHAKE

Servings: 1

Prep Time: 5 min

Total Time: 5 min

Ingredients:

- 1 cup of unsweetened almond milk
- ½ cup of frozen blueberries
- 1 scoop vanilla protein powder (sugar-free)
- 1 tbsp chia seeds
- ½ tsp vanilla extract

Instructions:

1. Blend the protein powder, chia seeds, almond milk, frozen blueberries, and vanilla extract.
2. Blend till creamy and smooth.
3. Transfer to a glass and serve right away.

Nutrition Info (per serving):

Calories: 180

Protein: 20g

Carbohydrates: 15g

Fat: 5g

Sodium: 110mg

Potassium: 200mg

CHAPTER 6: LUNCH RECIPES

1. GRILLED CHICKEN WITH HERB QUINOA SALAD

Servings: 4

Prep Time: 15 min

Cook Time: 20 min

Total Time: 35 min

Ingredients:

- 4 boneless, skinless chicken breasts
- 1 cup of quinoa, rinsed
- 2 cups of low-sodium chicken broth
- 1 tbsp olive oil
- 2 tbsp fresh parsley, chop-up
- 1 tbsp fresh mint, chop-up
- 1 tbsp lemon juice
- 1 tsp lemon zest
- 1 tsp garlic powder
- ¼ tsp black pepper

Instructions:

1. Set the grill's temperature to medium-high.
2. Use garlic powder and black pepper to season the chicken breasts. Grill for 6–7 minutes on every side.
3. Put the chicken stock in a saucepan until it boils. Reduce the heat, add the quinoa, cover, and After 15 mins or so, the liquid should be absorbed.
4. Using a fork, fluff the quinoa and mix in the lemon juice, lemon zest, parsley, and mint.
5. Serve the herb quinoa salad with the grilled chicken.

Nutrition Info (per serving):

Calories: 310

Protein: 35g

Carbohydrates: 22g

Fat: 8g

Sodium: 80mg

Potassium: 400mg

2. KIDNEY-FRIENDLY LENTIL SOUP

Servings: 6

Prep Time: 10 min

Cook Time: 40 min

Total Time: 50 min

Ingredients:

- 1 cup of dry lentils, rinsed
- 4 cups of low-sodium vegetable broth
- 1 medium carrot, diced
- 1 celery stalk, diced
- 1 small onion, chop-up
- 1 clove garlic, chop-up
- 1 tbsp olive oil
- 1 tsp dried thyme
- ¼ tsp black pepper

Instructions:

1. Flame the olive oil in a big pot over medium heat. For five to seven minutes, sauté the onion, carrot, celery, and garlic until tender.
2. Add the black pepper, thyme, lentils, and vegetable broth. After bringing it to a boil, lower the temperature and simmer the lentils for 30 to 35 min or until soft.
3. Serve hot, adjusting the seasoning if necessary.

Nutrition Info (per serving):

Calories: 180

Protein: 12g

Carbohydrates: 30g

Fat: 3g

Sodium: 90mg

Potassium: 300mg

3. VEGGIE WRAP WITH HUMMUS

Servings: 2

Prep Time: 10 min

Total Time: 10 min

Ingredients:

- 2 whole wheat tortillas
- ½ cup of hummus
- 1 small cucumber, split
- 1 small red bell pepper, split
- ½ cup of shredded lettuce
- ¼ cup of shredded carrots
- 2 tbsp crumbled feta cheese (non-compulsory)

Instructions:

1. Spread every tortilla with ¼ cup of hummus.
2. Arrange the carrots, lettuce, red bell pepper, and cucumber on the hummus.
3. If using, top with crumbled feta cheese.
4. Tightly roll the tortilla, cut it in half, and serve immediately.

Nutrition Info (per serving):

Calories: 220

Protein: 7g

Carbohydrates: 30g

Fat: 9g

Sodium: 200mg

Potassium: 320mg

4. BAKED SALMON WITH ROASTED VEGETABLES

Servings: 4

Prep Time: 10 min

Cook Time: 25 min

Total Time: 35 min

Ingredients:

- 4 salmon fillets (about 4-6 oz every)
- 1 tbsp olive oil
- 1 tsp lemon zest
- 1 tbsp lemon juice
- 1 tsp garlic powder
- 1 cup of broccoli florets
- 1 cup of diced zucchini
- 1 cup of diced bell peppers
- ¼ tsp black pepper

Instructions:

1. Set the oven's temperature to 375°F.
2. Line a sheet of pan with parchment paper and set the salmon fillets on top. Pour olive oil and lemon juice over the top, then top with garlic powder and lemon zest.
3. On the same sheet, arrange the bell peppers, broccoli, and zucchini around the salmon. Season with black pepper and drizzle the veggies with olive oil.
4. Bake for 20 to 25 minutes or until the fish is cooked and the vegetables tender.
5. Serve right away.

Nutrition Info (per serving):

Calories: 320

Protein: 30g

Carbohydrates: 12g

Fat: 18g

Sodium: 70mg

Potassium: 500mg

5. TURKEY AND ZUCCHINI LETTUCE WRAPS

Servings: 4

Prep Time: 15 min

Cook Time: 10 min

Total Time: 25 min

Ingredients:

- 1 lb lean ground turkey
- 1 zucchini, lightly diced
- 2 garlic cloves, chop-up
- 1 tbsp olive oil
- 1 tsp ground cumin
- 1 tsp smoked paprika
- 8 large lettuce leaves (for wrapping)
- 1 tbsp low-sodium soy sauce
- 1 tbsp fresh lime juice

Instructions:

1. In a skillet, Flame the olive oil over medium temperature. Cook, stirring occasionally, for 5–7 mins, or until browned, adding the ground turkey.
2. Add cumin, smoked paprika, diced zucchini, and garlic. Just a few more minutes of cooking should be enough to soften the zucchini.
3. With the lime juice and soy sauce added, mix well. Take off the heat.
4. Wrap the lettuce leaves after spooning the turkey mixture into them.
5. Serve right away.

Nutrition Info (per serving):

Calories: 220

Protein: 26g

Carbohydrates: 8g

Fat: 10g

Sodium: 150mg

Potassium: 320mg

6. GRILLED TOFU WITH SPINACH SALAD

Servings: 4

Prep Time: 15 min

Cook Time: 10 min

Total Time: 25 min

Ingredients:

1. 1 block firm tofu, drained and pressed
2. 1 tbsp olive oil
3. 1 tsp garlic powder
4. 1 tsp paprika
5. 6 cups of fresh spinach
6. 1 cup of cherry tomatoes, halved
7. ½ cucumber, split
8. 2 tbsp balsamic vinegar
9. 1 tbsp lemon juice

Instructions:

1. Turn the heat up to medium on a grill or grill pan.
2. Cut the tofu into slices that are 1 inch thick. Sprinkle with paprika and garlic powder after brushing both sides with olive oil.
3. The tofu should be golden brown after grilling for 4–5 min on every side.
4. Put the cucumber, cherry tomatoes, and spinach in a big bowl.
5. Whisk lemon juice and balsamic vinegar together. To coat, drizzle over the salad and toss.
6. Top the spinach salad with the grilled tofu.

Nutrition Info (per serving):

Calories: 180

Protein: 12g

Carbohydrates: 10g

Fat: 10g

Sodium: 70mg

Potassium: 450mg

7. QUINOA AND BLACK BEAN SALAD

Servings: 4

Prep Time: 10 min

Cook Time: 15 min

Total Time: 25 min

Ingredients:

- 1 cup of quinoa, rinsed
- 2 cups of water
- One cup of rinsed and drained canned black beans
- 1 cup of corn kernels
- ½ red bell pepper, diced
- ¼ cup of chop-up cilantro
- 2 tbsp olive oil
- 2 tbsp lime juice
- 1 tsp ground cumin
- ¼ tsp black pepper

Instructions:

1. In a medium pot, Put water to a boil. Reduce temperature to low, add the quinoa and cover. After 15 minutes of simmering, or until the water has been absorbed, the quinoa should be cooked.
2. Put the cooked quinoa, black beans, corn, cilantro, and red bell pepper in a big bowl.
3. Mix the lime juice, cumin, black pepper, and olive oil in a small bowl.
4. After adding the dressing to the quinoa mixture, toss to blend.
5. You can serve it cold or warm.

Nutrition Info (per serving):

Calories: 240

Protein: 8g

Carbohydrates: 38g

Fat: 7g

Sodium: 80mg

Potassium: 400mg

8. LOW-SODIUM TUNA SALAD

Servings: 2

Prep Time: 10 min

Total Time: 10 min

Ingredients:

- 1 can low-sodium tuna, drained
- 2 tbsp plain Greek yogurt
- 1 tsp Dijon mustard
- 1 tbsp lemon juice
- 1 celery stalk, diced
- ¼ small red onion, diced
- ¼ tsp black pepper
- 1 tbsp chop-up parsley

Instructions:

1. Mix the tuna, Greek yogurt, lemon juice, celery, red onion, Dijon mustard, and black pepper in a medium-sized bowl.
2. Stir thoroughly until adequately blended.
3. Before serving, scatter chop-up parsley on top.
4. Serve in lettuce wraps, over salad greens, or whole wheat toast.

Nutrition Info (per serving):

Calories: 150

Protein: 22g

Carbohydrates: 4g

Fat: 4g

Sodium: 70mg

Potassium: 280mg

9. CABBAGE SLAW WITH CHICKEN

Servings: 4

Prep Time: 15 min

Cook Time: 10 min (for chicken)

Total Time: 25 min

Ingredients:

- 2 cups of shredded cabbage
- 1 large carrot, shredded
- 1 bell pepper, thinly split
- 2 cups of cooked, shredded chicken breast
- 1 tbsp olive oil
- 2 tbsp apple cider vinegar
- 1 tbsp Dijon mustard
- 1 tsp honey (non-compulsory)
- ¼ tsp black pepper

Instructions:

1. Put the bell pepper, carrot, and shredded cabbage in a big bowl.
2. In the bowl, add the chicken shreds.
3. Combine the apple cider vinegar, honey (if using), Dijon mustard, olive oil, and black pepper in a small bowl and whisk to mix.
4. Cover the chicken and cabbage mixture with the dressing and toss to coat.
5. Serve cold or warm.

Nutrition Info (per serving):

Calories: 210

Protein: 25g

Carbohydrates: 12g

Fat: 8g

Sodium: 75mg

Potassium: 350mg

10. DIABETIC-FRIENDLY VEGETABLE STIR-FRY

Servings: 4

Prep Time: 10 min

Cook Time: 15 min

Total Time: 25 min

Ingredients:

- 1 tbsp olive oil
- 1 small onion, split
- 1 bell pepper, split
- 1 zucchini, split
- 1 cup of broccoli florets
- 1 cup of snap peas
- 1 tsp garlic powder
- 1 tbsp low-sodium soy sauce
- 1 tsp sesame oil
- 1 tbsp sesame seeds (non-compulsory)

Instructions:

1. In a large skillet, flame the olive oil over medium temperatures.
2. Include the slices of onion and bell pepper and cook for 3–4 minutes or until tender.
3. Add snap peas, broccoli, and zucchini. Cook until the vegetables are crisp but soft, for about 5 to 7 minutes.
4. Drizzle the vegetables with low-sodium soy sauce and sprinkle with garlic powder, mixing to mix.
5. Take off the heat and mix in the sesame oil.
6. Serve right away, garnished with sesame seeds if preferred.

Nutrition Info (per serving):

Calories: 130

Protein: 4g

Carbohydrates: 18g

Fat: 7g

Sodium: 120mg

Potassium: 350mg

CHAPTER 7: DINNER RECIPES

1. GARLIC AND HERB CHICKEN WITH STEAMED BROCCOLI

Servings: 4

Prep Time: 10 min

Cook Time: 15 min

Total Time: 25 min

Ingredients:

- 4 boneless, skinless chicken breasts
- 1 tbsp olive oil
- 2 cloves garlic, chop-up
- 1 tsp dried thyme
- 1 tsp dried rosemary
- 1 tbsp lemon juice
- 4 cups of broccoli florets
- ¼ tsp black pepper

Instructions:

1. In a skillet, flame the olive oil over medium temperatures. Sauté the garlic for one minute.
2. Add the chicken breasts, black pepper, rosemary, and thyme. Cook until cooked through and golden brown, 6–7 min per side.
3. Before serving, drizzle with lemon juice.
4. While the chicken cooks, steam the broccoli in a steamer basket for 4 to 5 minutes or until it is tender.
5. Serve steamed broccoli with the chicken.

Nutrition Info (per serving):

Calories: 250

Protein: 32g

Carbohydrates: 6g

Fat: 10g

Sodium: 60mg

Potassium: 450mg

2. LOW-SODIUM TURKEY CHILI

Servings: 6

Prep Time: 10 min

Cook Time: 45 min

Total Time: 55 min

Ingredients:

- 1 lb lean ground turkey
- 1 small onion, chop-up
- 1 bell pepper, diced
- 2 garlic cloves, chop-up
- 1 can (15 oz) no-salt-added diced tomatoes
- 1 can (15 oz) no-salt-added kidney beans, drained and rinsed
- 1 tbsp chili powder
- 1 tsp cumin
- 1 tsp paprika
- ¼ tsp black pepper
- 1 cup of low-sodium vegetable broth

Instructions:

1. In a large pot, brown the ground turkey over moderate temperatures for 5 to 7 minutes or until cooked.
2. Sauté the garlic, bell pepper, and onion for three to four minutes or until tender.
3. Add black pepper, paprika, cumin, and chili powder and stir.
4. Add kidney beans, vegetable broth, and diced tomatoes.
5. Put to a simmer and cook, stirring regularly, for 30 min.
6. If preferred, top with fresh cilantro and serve hot.

Nutrition Info (per serving):

Calories: 210

Protein: 22g

Carbohydrates: 18g

Fat: 6g

Sodium: 70mg

Potassium: 380mg

3. GRILLED TILAPIA WITH SPINACH AND CAULIFLOWER MASH

Servings: 4

Prep Time: 15 min

Cook Time: 20 min

Total Time: 35 min

Ingredients:

- 4 tilapia fillets
- 1 tbsp olive oil
- 1 tsp garlic powder
- 1 tbsp lemon juice
- 4 cups of fresh spinach
- 1 head cauliflower, chop-up
- 2 tbsp unsweetened almond milk
- 1 tbsp olive oil (for mash)
- ¼ tsp black pepper

Instructions:

1. Set the grill's temperature to medium. Sprinkle the tilapia fillets with black pepper and garlic powder after brushing them with olive oil.
2. The tilapia should be cooked through every side of the grill after 3–4 min.
3. In the meantime, steam the cauliflower for ten min or until it is soft. Add black pepper, olive oil, and almond milk and mash.
4. Sauté spinach in a skillet until it wilts, about 2 to 3 min.
5. Serve the sautéed spinach and cauliflower mash beside the tilapia.

Nutrition Info (per serving):

Calories: 250

Protein: 25g

Carbohydrates: 10g

Fat: 10g

Sodium: 55mg

Potassium: 500mg

4. ZUCCHINI NOODLES WITH PESTO CHICKEN

Servings: 4

Prep Time: 15 min

Cook Time: 10 min

Total Time: 25 min

Ingredients:

- 4 zucchini, spiralized into noodles
- 2 boneless, skinless chicken breasts, split
- 2 tbsp olive oil
- 2 tbsp homemade pesto
- 1 tbsp lemon juice
- ¼ tsp black pepper
- 1 tbsp finely grated Parmesan cheese (non-compulsory)

Instructions:

1. Within a skillet, Put 1 tablespoon of olive oil over medium temperature. After 5 to 6 mins, the slices of chicken should be cooked thoroughly and browned.
2. In the same skillet, toss the zucchini noodles with the leftover olive oil and cook for two to three min or until they are just beginning to soften.
3. Stir the zucchini noodles along with the pesto and lemon juice.
4. Top the pesto chicken with Parmesan cheese and serve it over the zucchini noodles if preferred.

Nutrition Info (per serving):

Calories: 220

Protein: 22g

Carbohydrates: 10g

Fat: 10g

Sodium: 75mg

Potassium: 450mg

5. BAKED COD WITH LEMON AND HERBS

Servings: 4

Prep Time: 10 min

Cook Time: 20 min

Total Time: 30 min

Ingredients:

- 4 cod fillets (4-6 oz every)
- 2 tbsp olive oil
- 1 tsp lemon zest
- 1 tbsp lemon juice
- 1 tbsp fresh parsley, chop-up
- 1 tbsp fresh dill, chop-up
- ¼ tsp black pepper

Instructions:

1. Set the oven's temperature to 375°F.
2. Place the fish fillets on a parchment paper-lined baking sheet.
3. Drizzle the fillets with lemon zest, lemon juice, and olive oil—season with black pepper, dill, and parsley.
4. The fish should be flaky and cooked through after 15 to 20 minutes in the oven.
5. Serve with a simple salad or a side of steaming vegetables.

Nutrition Info (per serving):

Calories: 200

Protein: 25g

Carbohydrates: 3g

Fat: 9g

Sodium: 60mg

Potassium: 450mg

6. DIABETIC-FRIENDLY VEGGIE STIR-FRY

Servings: 4

Prep Time: 10 min

Cook Time: 15 min

Total Time: 25 min

Ingredients:

- 1 tbsp olive oil
- 1 small onion, split
- 1 bell pepper, split
- 1 zucchini, split
- 1 cup of broccoli florets
- 1 cup of snap peas
- 1 tsp garlic powder
- 1 tbsp low-sodium soy sauce
- 1 tsp sesame oil
- 1 tbsp sesame seeds (non-compulsory)

Instructions:

1. In a large skillet, flame the olive oil over medium temperatures.
2. Sauté the bell pepper and onion for three to four minutes or until tender.
3. Cook the snap peas, broccoli, and zucchini for five to seven more minutes or until crisp but still soft.
4. Combine garlic powder with low-sodium soy sauce and drizzle over the top. Mix to blend.
5. Remove the pan from the temperature and pour some sesame oil over it. Toss in some sesame seeds for garnish if you like.
6. Serve right away.

Nutrition Info (per serving):

Calories: 150

Protein: 5g

Carbohydrates: 18g

Fat: 7g

Sodium: 120mg

Potassium: 350mg

7. SEARED TOFU WITH MIXED VEGETABLES

Servings: 4

Prep Time: 10 min

Cook Time: 15 min

Total Time: 25 min

Ingredients:

- 1 block firm tofu, drained and pressed
- 1 tbsp olive oil
- 1 tsp garlic powder
- 1 tsp ground ginger
- 1 tbsp low-sodium soy sauce
- 1 cup of bell peppers, split
- 1 cup of snow peas
- 1 carrot, thinly split
- 2 tbsp sesame oil

Instructions:

1. Cut the tofu into one-inch cubes. Flame the olive oil in a pan over medium-high heat.
2. Tofu cubes should be added and seared for 3–4 min on every side or until golden brown.
3. After taking the tofu out of the pan, set it aside.
4. Add the ginger, garlic powder, and soy sauce to the same pan. Then, cook the bell peppers, carrots, and snow peas for 4–5 minutes or until crisp-tender.
5. Put the tofu back in the skillet and gently stir it with the veggies.
6. Serve hot, drizzled with sesame oil.

Nutrition Info (per serving):

Calories: 200

Protein: 15g

Carbohydrates: 18g

Fat: 12g

Sodium: 150mg

Potassium: 450mg

8. BAKED PORK CHOPS WITH ROASTED ROOT VEGETABLES

Servings: 4

Prep Time: 15 min

Cook Time: 40 min

Total Time: 55 min

Ingredients:

- 4 bone-in pork chops
- 1 tbsp olive oil
- 1 tsp garlic powder
- 1 tsp dried thyme
- 1 tsp paprika
- 2 medium carrots, chop-up
- 2 parsnips, chop-up
- 1 sweet potato, peeled and cubed
- 1 tbsp fresh rosemary, chop-up

Instructions:

1. Set the oven's temperature to 400°F.
2. Apply a mixture of olive oil, black pepper, paprika, thyme, and garlic powder to the pork chops.
3. Arrange the chop-up root vegetables (sweet potatoes, parsnips, and carrots) around the pork chops on a baking sheet.
4. Sprinkle the veggies with rosemary and drizzle them with olive oil.
5. After 30 to 35 minutes of roasting, the pork chops should be cooked through (internal temperature of 145°F), and the veggies should be soft.
6. Roasted root vegetables should be served alongside the pork chops.

Nutrition Info (per serving):

Calories: 350

Protein: 30g

Carbohydrates: 30g

Fat: 14g

Sodium: 75mg

Potassium: 800mg

9. LOW-POTASSIUM BEEF STIR-FRY

Servings: 4

Prep Time: 10 min

Cook Time: 12 min

Total Time: 22 min

Ingredients:

- 1 lb lean beef (sirloin or flank steak), thinly split
- 1 tbsp olive oil
- 1 small onion, split
- 1 cup of bell peppers, split
- 1 cup of snow peas
- 2 garlic cloves, chop-up
- 1 tbsp low-sodium soy sauce
- 1 tbsp rice vinegar
- 1 tsp cornstarch (non-compulsory for thickening)

Instructions:

1. In a large skillet, Flame the olive oil over medium-high heat. Cook the beef for four to five minutes or until it is browned.
2. After adding the onion, bell peppers, snow peas, and garlic, cook for three to four minutes or until the veggies are soft.
3. Combine soy sauce and rice vinegar and mix well. To make a thicker sauce, whisk together a little water and cornstarch in a saucepan.
4. Keep cooking for another minute or two until the sauce becomes thick.
5. Serve right away over a bed of greens or brown rice.

Nutrition Info (per serving):

Calories: 280

Protein: 25g

Carbohydrates: 15g

Fat: 14g

Sodium: 150mg

Potassium: 450mg

10. LENTIL AND VEGGIE STEW

Servings: 6

Prep Time: 10 min

Cook Time: 40 min

Total Time: 50 min

Ingredients:

- 1 cup of dried lentils, rinsed
- 1 tbsp olive oil
- 1 onion, chop-up
- 2 carrots, chop-up
- 2 celery stalks, chop-up
- 1 zucchini, chop-up
- 1 can (14.5 oz) no-salt-added diced tomatoes
- 4 cups of low-sodium vegetable broth
- 1 tsp ground cumin
- ½ tsp black pepper

Instructions:

1. In a large pot, flame the olive oil over a medium-high temperature. Add zucchini, celery, carrots, and onion. The vegetables should be softened after 5 to 7 min of sautéing.
2. Add the cumin, black pepper, diced tomatoes, vegetable broth, and rinsed lentils.
3. After bringing the mixture to a boil, lower the temperature and simmer it for 30 to 35 min or until the lentils are soft.
4. If desired, serve hot, topped with a dollop of low-fat yogurt or fresh parsley.

Nutrition Info (per serving):

Calories: 220

Protein: 12g

Carbohydrates: 40g

Fat: 5g

Sodium: 140mg

Potassium: 550mg

CHAPTER 8: SNACKS AND SMALL BITES

1. CUCUMBER AND HUMMUS BITES

Servings: 4

Prep Time: 10 min

Cook Time: 0 min

Total Time: 10 min

Ingredients:
- 1 cucumber, split into rounds
- ½ cup of hummus (low-sodium)
- 1 tbsp fresh parsley, chop-up
- 1 tbsp sesame seeds (non-compulsory)

Instructions:
1. Cut the cucumber into rounds that are ¼ inch thick.
2. Put a little hummus on every slice of cucumber.
3. Sesame seeds and chop-up parsley are non-compulsory garnishes.
4. Serve right away as a fabulous appetizer or snack.

Nutrition Info (per serving):

Calories: 100

Protein: 3g

Carbohydrates: 10g

Fat: 6g

Sodium: 50mg

Potassium: 250mg

2. LOW-SODIUM ALMONDS AND BERRIES

Servings: 4

Prep Time: 5 min

Cook Time: 0 min

Total Time: 5 min

Ingredients:
- ¼ cup of unsalted almonds
- 1 cup of mixed fresh berries (blueberries, strawberries, raspberries)
- 1 tbsp chia seeds (non-compulsory)

Instructions:
1. Almonds should be put in a small bowl.
2. Fill the bowl with the fresh berries.
3. If desired, top with chia seeds.
4. Serve as a side dish or as a quick and healthful snack.

Nutrition Info (per serving):

Calories: 200

Protein: 7g

Carbohydrates: 20g

Fat: 12g

Sodium: 0mg

Potassium: 350mg

3. ROASTED CHICKPEAS

Servings: 4

Prep Time: 10 min

Cook Time: 25 min

Total Time: 35 min

Ingredients:

- 1 can (15 oz) no-salt-added chickpeas, drained and rinsed
- 1 tbsp olive oil
- 1 tsp paprika
- ½ tsp garlic powder
- ¼ tsp black pepper

Instructions:

1. Set the oven's temperature to 400°F.
2. Apply a paper towel to the chickpeas to pat them dry.
3. Add the black pepper, garlic powder, paprika, and olive oil to the chickpeas.
4. Put them in a single layer on a baking pan.
5. Roast until crispy, tossing halfway through, 25 min.
6. Before serving, allow to cool.

Nutrition Info (per serving):

Calories: 160

Protein: 7g

Carbohydrates: 22g

Fat: 6g

Sodium: 0mg

Potassium: 400mg

4. NO-BAKE ENERGY BITES

Servings: 12

Prep Time: 10 min

Cook Time: 0 min

Total Time: 10 min

Ingredients:

- 1 cup of old-fashioned oats
- ½ cup of natural peanut butter
- ¼ cup of honey
- 2 tbsp chia seeds
- ¼ cup of ground flaxseeds
- ¼ cup of unsweetened shredded coconut

Instructions:

1. In a big bowl, combine the oats, peanut butter, honey, chia seeds, flaxseeds, and shredded coconut.
2. Stir until all ingredients are well mixed.
3. Create twelve bite-sized balls by rolling the mixture.
4. Set in the fridge for half an hr.
5. Keep in the refrigerator for up to a week in an airtight container.

Nutrition Info (per serving):

Calories: 120

Protein: 4g

Carbohydrates: 14g

Fat: 7g

Sodium: 5mg

Potassium: 120mg

5. DIABETIC-FRIENDLY GREEK YOGURT PARFAIT

Servings: 4

Prep Time: 5 min

Cook Time: 0 min

Total Time: 5 min

Ingredients:

- 2 cups of plain Greek yogurt (unsweetened)
- ½ cup of mixed berries (strawberries, blueberries, raspberries)
- 1 tbsp chia seeds
- 1 tbsp unsweetened almond butter
- 1 tbsp slivered almonds (non-compulsory)

Instructions:

1. Arrange the mixed berries and Greek yogurt in dishes or serving glasses.
2. Top with a drizzle of almond butter.
3. For crunch, you can add split almonds and chia seeds that are non-compulsory.
4. Serve right away or chill for up to two hrs.

Nutrition Info (per serving):

Calories: 180

Protein: 15g

Carbohydrates: 18g

Fat: 8g

Sodium: 30mg

Potassium: 350mg

6. CARROT AND CELERY STICKS WITH PEANUT BUTTER

Servings: 4

Prep Time: 5 min

Cook Time: 0 min

Total Time: 5 min

Ingredients:

- Four large carrots, sliced into sticks after peeling
- 4 celery stalks cut into sticks
- ¼ cup of natural peanut butter (unsweetened, no salt)

Instructions:

1. Cut the carrots into sticks after washing and peeling them.
2. Clean the celery stalks and chop them into sticks.
3. Accompany the carrot and celery sticks with peanut butter on the side for dipping.

Nutrition Info (per serving):

Calories: 150

Protein: 6g

Carbohydrates: 15g

Fat: 9g

Sodium: 0mg

Potassium: 450mg

7. HOMEMADE KALE CHIPS

Servings: 4

Prep Time: 10 min

Cook Time: 15 min

Total Time: 25 min

Ingredients:

- One bunch of kale, with the stems cut off and the leaves ripped into little pieces
- 1 tbsp olive oil
- 1 tsp garlic powder
- 1 tsp paprika
- Salt as needed

Instructions:

1. Set the oven's temperature to 350°F.
2. Thoroughly wash and pat the kale leaves.
3. Add paprika, garlic powder, olive oil, and salt to the kale.
4. Spread the greens out evenly on a baking pan.
5. Bake until crispy, flipping halfway through, 12 to 15 min.
6. Before serving, allow to cool.

Nutrition Info (per serving):

Calories: 70

Protein: 3g

Carbohydrates: 8g

Fat: 4g

Sodium: 30mg

Potassium: 300mg

8. HARD-BOILED EGGS WITH PEPPER

Servings: 4

Prep Time: 5 min

Cook Time: 10 min

Total Time: 15 min

Ingredients:

- 8 large eggs
- Ground black pepper as needed

Instructions:

1. Put the eggs in a pot and add water to cover them.
2. Bring to a boil over high temperature, then lower the heat and simmer for nine to ten minutes.
3. Take off the heat and let the eggs cool in ice water.
4. Add ground black pepper, cut the eggs in half, and peel them.
5. Serve right away.

Nutrition Info (per serving):

Calories: 78

Protein: 6g

Carbohydrates: 1g

Fat: 5g

Sodium: 60mg

Potassium: 60mg

9. COTTAGE CHEESE WITH PEACHES (NO SUGAR)

Servings: 4

Prep Time: 5 min

Cook Time: 0 min

Total Time: 5 min

Ingredients:

- 1 cup of low-fat cottage cheese
- 1 fresh peach, split (or ½ cup of no-sugar-added canned peaches)

Instructions:

1. Fill every bowl with ¼ cup of cottage cheese.
2. Add fresh peach slices on top.
3. Serve right away as a light dinner or nutritious snack.

Nutrition Info (per serving):

Calories: 120

Protein: 12g

Carbohydrates: 14g

Fat: 2g

Sodium: 220mg

Potassium: 270mg

10. ALMOND FLOUR CRACKERS WITH GUACAMOLE

Servings: 4

Prep Time: 15 min

Cook Time: 10 min

Total Time: 25 min

Ingredients:

- 1 cup of almond flour
- 1 egg
- ½ tsp garlic powder
- ½ tsp dried rosemary
- ½ tsp salt
- 1 ripe avocado
- 1 tbsp lime juice
- 2 tbsp chop-up cilantro

Instructions:

1. Turn the oven on to 350°F.
2. Start by combining almond flour, egg, salt, rosemary, and garlic powder in a bowl. Mix until a dough forms.
3. To thin the dough, roll it between two sheets of parchment paper.
4. Slice into tiny squares or other shapes, then cook for 8 to 10 min.
5. Add the lime juice, cilantro, and salt after mashing the avocado in a bowl for the guacamole.
6. Present the crackers alongside the guacamole.

Nutrition Info (per serving):

Calories: 180

Protein: 6g

Carbohydrates: 9g

Fat: 14g

Sodium: 250mg

Potassium: 350mg

CHAPTER 9: DESSERTS

1. SUGAR-FREE APPLE CRISP

Servings: 6

Prep Time: 15 min

Cook Time: 40 min

Total Time: 55 min

Ingredients:

- 4 medium apples, peeled, cored, and split
- 1 tbsp lemon juice
- 1 tsp cinnamon
- 1 cup of rolled oats
- ¼ cup of almond flour
- ¼ cup of chop-up walnuts
- 2 tbsp melted coconut oil
- 1 tsp vanilla extract
- Stevia or monk fruit sweetener as needed

Instructions:

1. Set the oven's temperature to 350°F.
2. Arrange the apple slices in an oiled baking pan and toss them with cinnamon and lemon juice.
3. Oats, almond flour, walnuts, melted coconut oil, vanilla, and sweeteners should all be mixed in a separate bowl and stirred thoroughly.
4. On top of the apples, sprinkle the oat mixture.
5. Bake for 35 to 40 minutes until the apples are tender and the top is golden.
6. Serve warm and top with a dollop of yogurt or sugar-free whipped cream, if desired.

Nutrition Info (per serving):

Calories: 220

Protein: 4g

Carbohydrates: 27g

Fat: 12g

Sodium: 5mg

Potassium: 210mg

2. CHIA PUDDING WITH ALMOND MILK

Servings: 4

Prep Time: 5 min

Cook Time: 0 min

Total Time: 5 min (+ overnight refrigeration)

Ingredients:

- 1 cup of unsweetened almond milk
- 3 tbsp chia seeds
- 1 tsp vanilla extract
- 1-2 tbsp stevia or monk fruit sweetener
- Fresh berries or split almonds (non-compulsory)

Instructions:

1. Mix the chia seeds, almond milk, sugar, and vanilla in a bowl.
2. To avoid clumping, let it settle for five minutes and then mix again.
3. Refrigerate for at least three hrs or overnight, covered.
4. If preferred, garnish with split almonds or fresh berries before serving.

Nutrition Info (per serving):

Calories: 90

Protein: 2g

Carbohydrates: 8g

Fat: 6g

Sodium: 90mg

Potassium: 90mg

3. BAKED PEARS WITH CINNAMON

Servings: 4

Prep Time: 5 min

Cook Time: 20 min

Total Time: 25 min

Ingredients:

- 4 pears, halved and cored
- 1 tsp cinnamon
- 1 tbsp honey or sweetener of choice (non-compulsory)
- ¼ cup of chop-up pecans or walnuts (non-compulsory)

Instructions:

1. Set the oven's temperature to 375°F.
2. Put the cut side of the pear halves up on a baking tray.
3. Drizzle with honey (if used) and sprinkle with cinnamon.
4. Bake until the pears are soft, 20 to 25 min.
5. If desired, sprinkle chop-up nuts on top. Warm up and serve.

Nutrition Info (per serving):

Calories: 120

Protein: 1g

Carbohydrates: 31g

Fat: 2g

Sodium: 0mg

Potassium: 250mg

4. FROZEN BERRY YOGURT

Servings: 4

Prep Time: 5 min

Cook Time: 0 min

Total Time: 5 min (+ freezing time)

Ingredients:

- 2 cups of frozen mixed berries
- 1 cup of plain Greek yogurt (unsweetened)
- 1 tbsp honey or sweetener of choice (non-compulsory)
- 1 tsp vanilla extract

Instructions:

1. Blend the Greek yogurt, frozen berries, honey (if using), and vanilla extract.
2. Blend till creamy and smooth.
3. After transferring to a container, freeze for a minimum of two hrs.
4. After scooping, serve chilled.

Nutrition Info (per serving):

Calories: 120

Protein: 9g

Carbohydrates: 20g

Fat: 3g

Sodium: 40mg

Potassium: 230mg

5. LOW-CARB PUMPKIN BARS

Servings: 12

Prep Time: 10 min

Cook Time: 25 min

Total Time: 35 min

Ingredients:

- 1 cup of almond flour
- 1 tsp baking powder
- ½ tsp cinnamon
- ¼ tsp nutmeg
- ¼ tsp ginger
- 1 cup of canned pumpkin puree
- 3 large eggs
- ¼ cup of coconut oil, melted
- 1-2 tbsp stevia or monk fruit sweetener

Instructions:

1. Raise the oven to 350°F and coat a baking pan with oil.
2. Put the almond flour, baking powder, ginger, nutmeg, and cinnamon in a big basin.
3. Whisk the eggs, sweetener melted coconut oil, and pumpkin puree in a separate bowl.
4. Combine the dry and wet components and stir until a smooth mixture is achieved.
5. After the pan is ready, pour the batter and level it out.
6. After 25 to 30 minutes in the oven, remove the toothpick from the middle.
7. After cooling, cut into bars.

Nutrition Info (per serving):

Calories: 160

Protein: 6g

Carbohydrates: 8g

Fat: 14g

Sodium: 45mg

Potassium: 200mg

6. SUGAR-FREE CHOCOLATE MOUSSE

Servings: 4

Prep Time: 10 min

Cook Time: 0 min

Total Time: 10 min (+ refrigeration)

Ingredients:

- 1 cup of heavy whipping cream
- 2 tbsp unsweetened cocoa powder
- 1 tsp vanilla extract
- 2-3 tbsp stevia or monk fruit sweetener
- 1 tbsp unsweetened almond milk

Instructions:

1. Form soft peaks by whisking the heavy cream in a basin with a hand mixer.
2. Mix the cocoa powder, vanilla extract, and sweetener in a small bowl.
3. Add the almond milk and cocoa mixture to the whipped cream a little at a time and keep beating until everything is well blended and stiff peaks form.
4. Before serving, divide the mousse into serving dishes and refrigerate for at least an hour.

Nutrition Info (per serving):

Calories: 180

Protein: 2g

Carbohydrates: 4g

Fat: 17g

Sodium: 25mg

Potassium: 80mg

7. DIABETIC-FRIENDLY OATMEAL COOKIES

Servings: 12

Prep Time: 10 min

Cook Time: 15 min

Total Time: 25 min

Ingredients:

- 1 cup of rolled oats
- 1 cup of almond flour
- 1 tsp cinnamon
- ½ tsp baking soda
- 1 egg
- ¼ cup of unsweetened applesauce
- 1 tsp vanilla extract
- ¼ cup of stevia or monk fruit sweetener
- ½ cup of chop-up walnuts (non-compulsory)

Instructions:

1. Arrange parchment paper on a baking pan and set the oven temperature to 350°F.
2. Oats, almond flour, baking soda, and cinnamon should all be mixed in a bowl.
3. Whisk the egg, applesauce, vanilla, and sugar in another bowl.
4. Stir to mix the wet ingredients into the dry components.
5. If using, fold in chop-up walnuts.
6. Spoon dough onto the prepared baking sheet, then gently press to flatten.
7. Bake until golden brown, 12 to 15 min.
8. Before serving, allow to cool.

Nutrition Info (per serving):

Calories: 120

Protein: 4g

Carbohydrates: 10g

Fat: 9g

Sodium: 50mg

Potassium: 80mg

8. LEMON AND ALMOND CAKE

Servings: 8

Prep Time: 10 min

Cook Time: 30 min

Total Time: 40 min

Ingredients:

- 2 cups of almond flour
- 1 tsp baking powder
- ¼ tsp salt
- 3 large eggs
- ¼ cup of stevia or monk fruit sweetener
- ¼ cup of unsweetened almond milk
- 2 tbsp lemon zest
- 1 tsp vanilla extract

Instructions:

1. Put some butter in a cake pan and set the oven to 350˚F.
2. Salt, baking soda, and almond flour should be mixed together in a basin.
3. Whisk the eggs, almond milk, sugar, vanilla, and lemon zest in another bowl.
4. Mix the dry ingredients with the wet components until everything is well blended.
5. After the cake pan is ready, pour the batter into it.
6. After 25 to 30 minutes in the oven, remove the toothpick from the middle.
7. Before serving, let it cool.

Nutrition Info (per serving):

Calories: 190

Protein: 7g

Carbohydrates: 8g

Fat: 15g

Sodium: 60mg

Potassium: 120mg

9. LOW-SUGAR STRAWBERRY GELATIN

Servings: 4

Prep Time: 5 min

Cook Time: 5 min

Total Time: 10 min (+ refrigeration)

Ingredients:

- 1 cup of fresh strawberries, pureed
- 1 cup of water
- 1 tbsp gelatin powder (unsweetened)
- 2-3 tbsp stevia or monk fruit sweetener

Instructions:

1. Put the gelatin and water in a saucepan. Stir continuously while heating over medium temperature until the gelatin melts.
2. Stir in the sweetener and the pureed strawberries. Mix to blend.
3. After pouring the gelatin mixture into serving dishes, let it set in the refrigerator for at least two hrs.
4. Serve cold.

Nutrition Info (per serving):

Calories: 25

Protein: 1g

Carbohydrates: 5g

Fat: 0g

Sodium: 5mg

Potassium: 50mg

10. VANILLA ALMOND PUDDING

Servings: 4

Prep Time: 5 min

Cook Time: 10 min

Total Time: 15 min (+ refrigeration)

Ingredients:

- 2 cups of unsweetened almond milk
- 1 tbsp cornstarch
- 1 tsp vanilla extract
- 1 tbsp stevia or monk fruit sweetener
- 2 tbsp almond butter

Instructions:

1. Mix the cornstarch and almond milk in a saucepan. Whisk continuously while cooking over medium heat until the mixture thickens.
2. Add almond butter, sweetener, and vanilla extract. Mix until it's smooth.
3. Transfer to serving dishes and chill for at least one hr to ensure it solidifies.
4. Serve cold, with split almonds on top if desired.

Nutrition Info (per serving):

Calories: 120

Protein: 3g

Carbohydrates: 8g

Fat: 10g

Sodium: 50mg

Potassium: 150mg

CHAPTER 10: DRINKS AND SMOOTHIES

1. LOW-SUGAR GREEN SMOOTHIE

Servings: 2

Prep Time: 5 min

Cook Time: 0 min

Total Time: 5 min

Ingredients:

- 1 cup of spinach
- ½ cucumber, split
- ½ green apple, cored and split
- 1 tbsp chia seeds
- 1 cup of unsweetened almond milk
- 1 tbsp lemon juice
- Stevia or monk fruit sweetener as needed (non-compulsory)

Instructions:

1. Fill a blender with all the ingredients.
2. If additional almond milk is required to achieve the appropriate consistency, add it after blending until smooth and creamy.
3. If desired, add sweetener after tasting.
4. If preferred, top with a lemon wedge and serve right away.

Nutrition Info (per serving):

Calories: 50

Protein: 2g

Carbohydrates: 7g

Fat: 3g

Sodium: 50mg

Potassium: 300mg

2. HERBAL ICED TEA

Servings: 4

Prep Time: 5 min

Cook Time: 10 min

Total Time: 15 min (+ chilling)

Ingredients:

- 4 cups of water
- 4 herbal tea bags (chamomile, peppermint, or your choice)
- 1-2 tbsp stevia or monk fruit sweetener (non-compulsory)
- Ice cubes
- Lemon slices for garnish

Instructions:

1. In a saucepan, boil four cups of water.
2. Put the herbal tea bags in and let them brew for five to seven minutes.
3. Remove tea bags, let the tea cool to room temperature, and whisk in sweetener if preferred.
4. Refrigerate for one to two hrs.
5. Accompany with a sprig of lemon and serve chilled over ice.

Nutrition Info (per serving):

Calories: 5

Protein: 0g

Carbohydrates: 1g

Fat: 0g

Sodium: 0mg

Potassium: 20mg

3. DIABETIC-FRIENDLY LEMONADE

Servings: 4

Prep Time: 5 min

Cook Time: 0 min

Total Time: 5 min

Ingredients:

- 1 cup of fresh lemon juice
- 4 cups of water
- 1-2 tbsp stevia or monk fruit sweetener
- Ice cubes
- Lemon slices for garnish

Instructions:

1. Put water and fresh lemon juice in a pitcher.
2. To dissolve the sweetener, add it and stir.
3. Chill in the refrigerator for one hr.
4. Before serving over ice, garnish with lemon slices.

Nutrition Info (per serving):

Calories: 5

Protein: 0g

Carbohydrates: 2g

Fat: 0g

Sodium: 5mg

Potassium: 30mg

4. ALMOND MILK BERRY SMOOTHIE

Servings: 2

Prep Time: 5 min

Cook Time: 0 min

Total Time: 5 min

Ingredients:

- 1 cup of unsweetened almond milk
- ½ cup of mixed berries (blueberries, raspberries, strawberries)
- 1 tbsp almond butter
- ½ tsp vanilla extract
- Stevia or monk fruit sweetener as needed (non-compulsory)

Instructions:

1. Put everything in a blender.
2. Blend till creamy and smooth.
3. If desired, add sweetener after tasting.
4. Garnish with a few additional berries and serve right away.

Nutrition Info (per serving):

Calories: 90

Protein: 3g

Carbohydrates: 12g

Fat: 5g

Sodium: 40mg

Potassium: 150mg

5. SUGAR-FREE CHIA WATER

Servings: 2

Prep Time: 5 min

Cook Time: 0 min

Total Time: 5 min (+ chilling)

Ingredients:

- 2 cups of water
- 1 tbsp chia seeds
- 1-2 tbsp fresh lemon juice
- Stevia fruit sweetener as needed (non-compulsory)

Instructions:

1. Put the chia seeds and water in a pitcher or jar.
2. To let the chia seeds absorb the water and develop a gel-like consistency, stir them well and place them in the refrigerator for at least half an hr.
3. If desired, add sugar and lemon juice.
4. Before drinking, mix thoroughly and serve cold.

Nutrition Info (per serving):

Calories: 20

Protein: 1g

Carbohydrates: 4g

Fat: 1g

Sodium: 10mg

Potassium: 40mg

6. LOW-POTASSIUM CUCUMBER MINT COOLER

Servings: 2

Prep Time: 5 min

Cook Time: 0 min

Total Time: 5 min

Ingredients:

- 1 cucumber, peeled and split
- 6-8 fresh mint leaves
- 1 tbsp fresh lime juice
- 1-2 tbsp stevia or monk fruit sweetener
- 2 cups of cold water
- Ice cubes

Instructions:

1. Put the cucumber, lime juice, mint leaves, and sweetener in a blender.
2. Blend in cold water until smooth.
3. Pulp can be non-compulsorily removed by straining the mixture through a fine mesh screen.
4. Top with ice and serve right away.

Nutrition Info (per serving):

Calories: 10

Protein: 1g

Carbohydrates: 3g

Fat: 0g

Sodium: 5mg

Potassium: 120mg

7. WATERMELON AND BASIL SLUSHIE

Servings: 2

Prep Time: 5 min

Cook Time: 0 min

Total Time: 5 min

Ingredients:

- 2 cups of cubed watermelon
- 5-6 fresh basil leaves
- 1 tbsp lime juice
- 1 tbsp stevia or monk fruit sweetener
- Ice cubes

Instructions:

1. Mix the watermelon, sugar, lime juice, and basil in a blender.
2. Process until slushy and smooth.
3. To achieve the required consistency, add ice cubes and mix once more.
4. If preferred, top with additional basil leaves and serve right away.

Nutrition Info (per serving):

Calories: 45

Protein: 1g

Carbohydrates: 12g

Fat: 0g

Sodium: 10mg

Potassium: 150mg

8. ICED HERBAL TEA WITH LEMON

Servings: 4

Prep Time: 5 min

Cook Time: 5 min

Total Time: 10 min (+ chilling)

Ingredients:

- 4 cups of water
- 4 herbal tea bags (chamomile, peppermint, or your choice)
- 1-2 tbsp stevia or monk fruit sweetener (non-compulsory)
- 1 lemon, thinly split
- Ice cubes

Instructions:

1. Cook four cups of water until it boils.
2. Steep for five to seven min after adding the tea bags.
3. Take out the tea bags and, if you want, stir in some sweetness.
4. After letting the tea drop to room temperature, chill it in the refrigerator for one to two hrs.
5. Before serving over ice, garnish with lemon slices.

Nutrition Info (per serving):

Calories: 5

Protein: 0g

Carbohydrates: 1g

Fat: 0g

Sodium: 0mg

Potassium: 20mg

9. DIABETIC-FRIENDLY COCOA DRINK

Servings: 2

Prep Time: 5 min

Cook Time: 5 min

Total Time: 10 min

Ingredients:

- 2 cups of unsweetened almond milk
- 2 tbsp unsweetened cocoa powder
- 1-2 tbsp stevia or monk fruit sweetener
- ½ tsp vanilla extract
- ¼ tsp ground cinnamon (non-compulsory)

Instructions:

1. Flame the almond milk in a small saucepan over medium heat.
2. Add vanilla essence, sweetener, and cocoa powder and stir.
3. Flame until the mixture is smooth and hot, whisking continuously.
4. Transfer into cups of garnish with cinnamon, and serve immediately.

Nutrition Info (per serving):

Calories: 50

Protein: 2g

Carbohydrates: 5g

Fat: 3g

Sodium: 45mg

Potassium: 150mg

10. UNSWEETENED APPLE AND CINNAMON PUNCH

Servings: 4

Prep Time: 5 min

Cook Time: 0 min

Total Time: 5 min

Ingredients:
- 2 cups of unsweetened apple juice
- 2 cups of cold water
- 1 cinnamon stick
- 1 tbsp lemon juice
- Ice cubes

Instructions:
1. Put the water, lemon juice, apple juice, and cinnamon stick in a pitcher.
2. To chill and infuse the flavors, stir thoroughly and place in the refrigerator for one hr.
3. Before serving, remove the cinnamon stick and serve over ice.

Nutrition Info (per serving):

Calories: 40

Protein: 0g

Carbohydrates: 10g

Fat: 0g

Sodium: 5mg

Potassium: 150mg

CHAPTER 11: 30-DAY MEAL PLAN

Day	Breakfast	Lunch	Dinner	Snack
1	Oatmeal with berries and almond milk	Grilled chicken salad with mixed greens	Baked salmon with steamed vegetables	Celery sticks with hummus
2	Scrambled eggs with spinach and a slice of whole-grain toast	Turkey and avocado wrap (low-sodium tortilla)	Grilled shrimp with quinoa and sautéed zucchini	Cucumber slices with tzatziki sauce
3	Greek yogurt with chia seeds and strawberries	Baked chicken breast with roasted sweet potatoes	Baked cod with steamed green beans and a side of brown rice	Small apple with peanut butter
4	Smoothie with unsweetened almond milk, spinach, and protein powder	Tuna salad with mixed greens and olive oil dressing	Stir-fried tofu with broccoli and bell peppers over quinoa	Carrot sticks with light ranch dressing
5	Whole-grain toast with avocado and poached egg	Grilled chicken with sautéed kale and quinoa	Turkey meatballs with zucchini noodles	Handful of mixed nuts (unsalted)
6	Cottage cheese with cucumber and tomato slices	Chicken and vegetable stir-fry with low-sodium soy sauce	Baked turkey breast with roasted carrots and cauliflower	1 small pear
7	Chia seed pudding with almond milk and a few slices of banana	Grilled fish tacos with cabbage slaw (using low-sodium tortilla)	Lemon-baked chicken with steamed asparagus	Small handful of almonds
8	Scrambled egg whites with tomatoes and spinach	Grilled vegetable and quinoa bowl with olive oil and lemon	Baked tilapia with sautéed green beans	Celery with almond butter
9	Smoothie with berries, kale, and unsweetened almond milk	Quinoa salad with cucumber, chickpeas, and olive oil dressing	Grilled steak with mashed cauliflower and sautéed spinach	1 small apple with cheese
10	Whole-grain toast with cottage cheese and strawberries	Chicken breast with roasted Brussels sprouts	Shrimp stir-fry with snow peas and brown rice	Cucumber slices with hummus
11	Oatmeal with chia seeds and blueberries	Turkey and avocado lettuce wraps	Grilled salmon with a side of roasted butternut squash	Carrot sticks with hummus

12	Greek yogurt with flaxseeds and raspberries	Chicken Caesar salad (use low-sodium dressing)	Baked chicken thighs with quinoa and steamed broccoli	Small handful of walnuts
13	Scrambled eggs with mushrooms and onions	Baked chicken breast with roasted vegetables	Grilled shrimp with mixed greens and olive oil dressing	1 small pear
14	Chia seed pudding with almond milk and strawberries	Grilled turkey breast with mixed vegetable salad	Stir-fried tofu with bok choy and brown rice	Small handful of mixed nuts
15	Whole-grain toast with avocado and egg	Tuna salad with mixed greens and olive oil dressing	Grilled chicken breast with roasted zucchini and quinoa	Carrot sticks with light ranch
16	Smoothie with unsweetened almond milk, kale, and protein powder	Grilled salmon with a side of mixed greens	Baked chicken with roasted sweet potatoes and steamed asparagus	Small apple with almond butter
17	Oatmeal with flaxseeds and strawberries	Quinoa salad with grilled chicken and mixed vegetables	Baked cod with sautéed spinach and quinoa	1 small pear
18	Scrambled egg whites with spinach and mushrooms	Chicken and vegetable stir-fry with quinoa	Grilled steak with steamed cauliflower and green beans	Small handful of almonds
19	Greek yogurt with chia seeds and raspberries	Grilled chicken with mixed vegetable salad	Stir-fried tofu with bell peppers and quinoa	Celery with peanut butter
20	Whole-grain toast with avocado and poached egg	Tuna salad with avocado and mixed greens	Grilled shrimp with roasted sweet potatoes	Cucumber slices with hummus
21	Chia seed pudding with almond milk and blueberries	Grilled turkey breast with roasted Brussels sprouts	Baked tilapia with a side of quinoa and steamed asparagus	Small handful of walnuts
22	Scrambled eggs with tomatoes and spinach	Grilled chicken with mixed vegetable salad	Lemon-baked chicken with steamed green beans	Carrot sticks with hummus
23	Smoothie with unsweetened almond milk, berries, and protein powder	Quinoa salad with chickpeas, cucumber, and olive oil	Stir-fried tofu with broccoli and bell peppers	Small apple with almond butter

24	Oatmeal with chia seeds and strawberries	Grilled chicken with quinoa and roasted vegetables	Grilled fish tacos with cabbage slaw (low-sodium tortilla)	Celery with hummus
25	Greek yogurt with flaxseeds and raspberries	Turkey and avocado wrap (low-sodium tortilla)	Baked salmon with steamed spinach and roasted carrots	Carrot sticks with light ranch
26	Scrambled egg whites with spinach and mushrooms	Grilled chicken with roasted cauliflower	Stir-fried shrimp with mixed vegetables and quinoa	Small handful of mixed nuts
27	Whole-grain toast with cottage cheese and cucumber	Grilled chicken breast with a side of roasted vegetables	Baked cod with sautéed spinach and quinoa	Small pear
28	Smoothie with almond milk, kale, and protein powder	Grilled salmon with mixed greens and olive oil dressing	Baked chicken with roasted sweet potatoes and steamed asparagus	Cucumber slices with hummus
29	Oatmeal with blueberries and chia seeds	Tuna salad with mixed greens and olive oil dressing	Stir-fried tofu with bok choy and brown rice	Carrot sticks with hummus
30	Greek yogurt with chia seeds and strawberries	Grilled turkey breast with roasted Brussels sprouts	Grilled chicken with quinoa and steamed broccoli	Small handful of almonds

CHAPTER 12: GROCERY SHOPPING LIST

Category	Item
Proteins	Chicken breasts (skinless, boneless)
	Chicken thighs (skinless, boneless)
	Turkey breast
	Ground turkey (lean)
	Salmon fillets
	Cod fillets
	Tilapia fillets
	Shrimp (fresh or frozen)
	Tofu (firm)
	Eggs (preferably organic or free-range)

	Egg whites (if preferred separately)
	Canned tuna (in water, low-sodium)
	Greek yogurt (plain, unsweetened)
	Cottage cheese (low-sodium)
Grains	Quinoa
	Brown rice
	Whole-grain bread (low-sodium)
	Whole-grain tortillas (low-sodium)
	Oats (old-fashioned or steel-cut)
	Whole-grain crackers (low-sodium)
Vegetables	Kale
	Spinach (fresh or frozen)
	Mixed salad greens (arugula, romaine, etc.)
	Broccoli (fresh or frozen)
	Zucchini
	Bell peppers (red, yellow, or green)
	Cucumbers
	Carrots
	Cauliflower
	Brussels sprouts
	Green beans
	Asparagus
	Sweet potatoes
	Mushrooms
	Tomatoes (in moderation)
	Snow peas
	Cabbage (for slaw)
	Bok choy
Fruits	Apples
	Pears
	Blueberries (fresh or frozen)
	Strawberries (fresh or frozen)
	Raspberries (fresh or frozen)

	Bananas (limited, if desired—moderate potassium)
Dairy & Dairy Alternatives	Unsweetened almond milk
	Low-sodium cheese (cheddar, mozzarella, or cream cheese)
Healthy Fats	Olive oil
	Avocados
	Almonds (unsalted)
	Walnuts (unsalted)
	Peanut butter (unsweetened, no added salt)
Legumes & Beans	Chickpeas (canned or dried, low-sodium)
	Black beans (canned or dried, low-sodium)
	Lentils (dried or canned, low-sodium)
Herbs & Spices	Fresh parsley
	Fresh basil
	Fresh thyme
	Fresh cilantro
	Garlic (fresh or minced)
	Ginger
	Black pepper
	Turmeric
	Cinnamon
	Oregano
	Cumin
	Paprika
	Red pepper flakes
	Lemon juice (fresh or bottled)
	Lime juice (fresh or bottled)
Condiments & Sauces	Low-sodium soy sauce
	Olive oil-based dressing (or make your own with olive oil, vinegar, and spices)
	Low-sodium mustard
	Balsamic vinegar
	Apple cider vinegar
	Hummus (low-sodium)

Snacks	Mixed nuts (unsalted)
	Unsweetened applesauce
	Low-sodium popcorn (for an occasional snack)
Frozen Items	Frozen spinach
	Frozen broccoli
	Frozen berries (strawberries, blueberries, raspberries)
Beverages	Herbal teas (chamomile, peppermint, etc.)
	Green tea
	Coffee (in moderation, with unsweetened almond milk if desired)
Additional Items (Optional)	Protein powder (unsweetened, plant-based or whey)
	Chia seeds
	Flaxseeds
	Stevia or monk fruit (as natural sweeteners)
	Sugar-free gelatin (as a low-sugar treat)
	Whole-grain granola (low-sodium, for topping yogurt)

THE END

Made in United States
Orlando, FL
17 July 2025